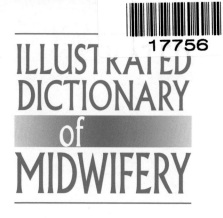

ILLUSTRATED
DICTIONARY
of
MIDWIFERY

To the memory of
Tim Winson,
friend,
husband and father.

For Elsevier:

Commissioning Editor: Mary Seager
Development Editor: Catharine Steers
Project Manager: Derek Robertson
Designer: George Ajayi

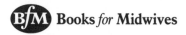
BfM Books *for* Midwives

ILLUSTRATED DICTIONARY
of
MIDWIFERY

Nicola V Winson MA PGCEA ADM RM RN
Senior Lecturer, Wolfson Institute, Thames Valley University

Sandra McDonald MSc Education
Senior Lecturer, Thames Valley University

ELSEVIER

Edinburgh London New York Oxford Philadelphia St Louis Sydney Toronto 2005

ELSEVIER

First published 2005
    Reprinted 2006

ISBN 0 7506 5327 2

British Library Cataloguing in Publication Data
A catalogue record for this book is available from the British Library

Library of Congress Cataloguing in Publication Data
A catalogue record for this book is available from the Library of Congress

Notice
Medical knowledge is constantly changing. Standard safety precautions must be followed, but as new research and clinical experience broaden our knowledge, changes in treatment and drug therapy may become necessary r appropriate. Readers are advised to check the most current product information provided by the manufacturer of each drug to be administered to verify the recommended dose, the method and duration of administration, and contraindications. It is the responsibility of the practitioner, relying on experience and knowledge of the patient, to determine dosages and the best treatment for each individual patient. Neither the Publisher nor the editors assume any liability for any injury and/or damage to persons or property arising from this publication.

The Publisher

Printed and bound in China

Contents

Preface

Midwives are very aware that they live in a rapidly changing world. The profession has responded with sensitivity and flexibility to the challenges and competing demands being made upon it from many directions: from women and their families, government, society, obstetricians and other health care professions. An indication of this has been the way midwives have expanded into areas of specialism to become consultants providing care to particularly needy groups of women such as those with HIV, diabetes and high risk pregnancy and entering the arena of public health. Further areas of diversification for midwives have been in the fields of management, research and education.

Committed men and women are being recruited to the career of midwifery and this dictionary is designed to help them appreciate the diversity of the profession they are joining and the scope available within it for their future growth. The illustrations are intended to aid understanding and provide a pointer towards more comprehensive texts where greater depth is required. It is anticipated that the dictionary will be of use to affiliated groups engaged in educating women for childbirth experiences, to women and to para-midwifery professions.

This reference book is dedicated to all those midwives who, over the years, have used their expertise to respond to the changing needs of women in the childbearing years. May their sensitivity and flexibility serve as an example to those who come after them.

Nicola Winson and Sandra McDonald
Senior Lecturers, Midwifery
Thames Valley University

Aa

abdomen (belly) the enclosed area beneath the diaphragm and above the pelvis containing the organs of digestion and the liver. The rectus muscle of the abdomen covers the anterior wall and is capable of great distension to accommodate the gravid uterus and distended bladder.

abdominal relating to the abdomen, for example *abdominal pregnancy* (*see* entry and Figure 1, below), where the embryo develops in the abdominal cavity.

abdominal adhesion the binding together by abnormal fibrous bands, sometimes causing pain and loss of movement. May occur following caesaean section or other surgical procedure.

abdominal breathing excessive movement of abdominal wall during respiration; often seen in neonates with immature lungs. Can be indicative of respiratory distress.

abdominal cavity the space between the diaphragm and the pelvic cavity lined by the peritoneum and containing the liver, gall bladder, intestines, stomach and spleen. Situated on the posterior abdominal wall and behind the peritoneum are the kidneys.

abdominal delivery birth of an infant through an incision into the abdominal wall and uterus; this includes caesarean section.

abdominal examination assessment of the abdomen using three senses, observation, palpation and auscultation; this is done during pregnancy to assess growth and detect possible abnormalities.

abdominal girth measurement of the abdominal circumference; may be carried out a number of times to detect rapid increase that may be diagnostic of polyhydramnios.

abdominal pain severe regional discomfort which inhibits normal activities causing the sufferer to seek midwifery or medical attention.

abdominal palpation the part of abdominal examination in which the operator feels the abdomen to detect resistance, or absence of resistance, indicating the size and position of internal contents.

abdominal pregnancy occurs where the embryo embeds itself outside the uterus, perhaps on the intestinal wall, and may grow to term (*see* Figure 1).

abdominal regions the division of the abdomen into named sectors in a three-by-three pattern (*see* Figure 2).

abduction the movement of individual parts of the body away from the mid-line.

abnormality a deviation from the usual or what is normal; a condition not found in the majority of individuals.

ABO blood grouping the genetically determined classification of human blood as determined by the presence or absence of antigens.

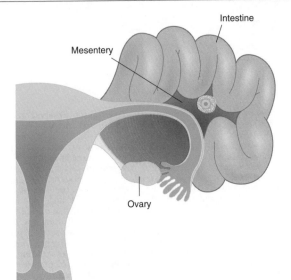

■ **Figure 1** Abdominal pregnancy

Group	Erythrocyte antigen (agglutinogen)	Serum antibody (agglutinin)
O	A and B absent	Anti-A and anti-B
A	A present	Anti-B present
B	B present	Anti-A present
AB	A and B present	No antibody present

ABO incompatibility this can occur where the maternal blood group is O, containing both anti-A and anti-B antibodies, and the fetus is of group A, group B or group AB. Transplacental crossing of maternal antibodies may lead to haemolysis of fetal erythrocytes in various degrees of severity, jaundice, anaemia, heart failure or death.

abort to end pregnancy before the 24th completed week.

abortifacient a drug or other substance used to induce an abortion.

abortion the induced termination of a pregnancy before the age of viability.

abortion on demand a service offered to women by which a pregnancy can be terminated at the woman's request.

abortus name given to the fetus that has been aborted.

abrasion superficial injury to tissue, usually as a result of trauma.

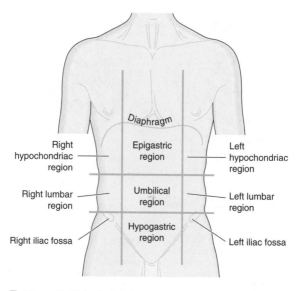

Right hypochondriac region

Epigastric region

Left hypochondriac region

Right lumbar region

Umbilical region

Left lumbar region

Hypogastric region

Right iliac fossa

Left iliac fossa

Diaphragm

■ **Figure 2** Abdominal regions

abruptio placentae accidental and premature separation of part or all of a normally situated placenta prior to delivery which results in bleeding that may be revealed, concealed or a combination of both (*see* Figure 3). Fetal distress may be mild or severe and may lead to intrauterine death.

abruption a tearing away.

abscess a local collection of pus. Abscess formation is not uncommon in the breast following acute mastitis. Other common sites are in the Bartholin's glands at the entrance to the vagina and in the pouch of Douglas.

absorb to soak up fluids or gases. Components are drawn into one another across a membrane, becoming a unified whole.

absorbable surgical suture material used to close an inci-

sion or wound which does not require removal.

absorption the ability of the body to engulf matter, fluids or gases into the circulatory system.

abstinence to go without; avoidance of or refraining from (e.g.) sexual intercourse.

abuse cruelty or mistreatment of one person by another.

acardia absence of a heart. This congenital condition is rarely seen now except in conjoined twins as it can be detected by ultrasound scan and termination of pregnancy offered.

acardius acephalus absence of heart, head and upper parts of the body.

accelerate (SYNONYM augment) to quicken, as in to *accelerate labour* or speed its progress by the use of drugs. Oxytocin is most commonly used.

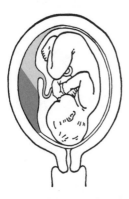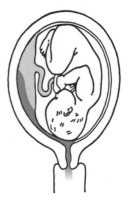

■ **Figure 3** Abruptio placentae

acceleration phase period of labour in which the greatest cervical dilation is achieved, between 3 and 10 cm.

accessory additional or supplementary, e.g. abdominal muscles are *accessories* to respiration and to pushing in the active second stage of labour.

accessory placenta placental tissue supplementary to the main organ and connected to it by blood vessels.

accoucheur a professionally trained person who attends women in childbirth; midwife or obstetrician.

accountability to answer for one's conduct; the requirement that a professional person accepts responsibility for and explains their independently performed actions upon request.

accreditation the acknowledgement of prior achievements.

accreta complete attachment, as in *placenta accreta*, where the placenta is deeply embedded, perhaps into the myometrium.

accretion adhesion of parts that are normally separate.

acephaly congenital absence of the head.

acetabulum a hemispherical depression situated on the lateral surface of the innominate bone (sides of the pelvis) into which fits the head of the femur (thigh bone).

acetone the smell on the breath or in the urine of a person who is using fat to make energy. The resulting ketone bodies may be secreted by the lungs.

achondrogenesis a type of dwarfism in which limbs and trunk are particularly shortened.

achondroplasia a genetically acquired disorder of bone growth, characterized by arrested growth of the long bones resulting in short stature or dwarfism. The head is large, trunk is of normal size and intellect is normal.

achromatic lacking in colour. Red blood cells may lack colour in certain types of anaemia.

acid–base balance the state of equilibrium existing in the body when the body fluids achieve their appropriate pH value, e.g. blood pH 7.4, gastric juices pH 2.3, urine pH 4–5, on the acid–alkaline continuum.

acid-fast bacillus classification of bacteria by their ability to hold an administered dye when its removal is attempted with acid.

acidaemia an accumulation of acid in the blood altering its predominantly alkaline state.

acidity degree of sharpness or sourness of taste; hydrogen ions are freely given out when dissolved in water.

acidity of the stomach relates to the acid–alkaline climate of the stomach. Inhalation of gastric juices during induction of anaesthesia causes burning of the lung – Mendelson's syndrome. An antacid may be offered in labour.

acidosis a state created by depletion of the body's alkaline reserve and disturbance of the acid–base balance. Results from the body metabolizing fat for energy instead of carbohydrate.

acini plural of acinus.

acinus a small hollow sac or lobule lined by secreting cells and containing a duct.

acme peak, height; most painful part of a uterine contraction.

acne inflammation or sepsis in small sebaceous glands in the skin; commonly occurring on the face, chest and back.

acne neonatorum small white spots seen on the infant's skin.

acquired not inherited, developed in response to intentional or environmental exposure.

acquired immune deficiency syndrome (AIDS) progressive disease caused by the human immunodeficiency virus (HIV) which reduces the body's response to infection and tumour formation. Death occurs due to generalized debility and an opportunistic infection or tumour. The virus can be passed to the fetus.

acquired immunity enhanced resistance of a host to disease by passive or active exposure stimulating antibodies to develop.

acquired sterility inability to conceive a second child.

acromial referring to the acromion.

acromion the triangular bony extension of the scapula which forms the point of the shoulder.

Act of Parliament the process by which an intended action passes through the lower and upper houses of parliament and receives royal assent to become law. (The first Midwives' Act of 1902 legalized midwifery and gave midwives the status of professionals.)

ACTH (adrenocorticotrophic hormone) hormone secreted by the anterior lobe of the pituitary gland, its target being the adrenal cortex where it stimulates the production of corticosteroids.

actinism the ability of sunlight and ultraviolet (UV) radiation to cause chemical changes in the skin. This occurs when jaundiced neonates are exposed to sunlight or UV light; the bile pigment in the skin is broken down.

active immunity resistance to disease resulting from exposure by infection or vaccination.

active labour the process by which strong contractions cause the cervix to dilate and the fetus to pass through the birth canal.

active listening a series of questions, nods and other nonverbal signs that a midwife uses to encourage parents to continue talking or clarifying their thoughts following an event or during decision making. An essential part of enabling informed choice.

active management of labour a process of intervention intended to prevent prolonged labour. It includes rupturing the membranes, accelerating labour with oxytocin and instrumental delivery. Active management of the third stage became normal procedure in the 1960s to reduce the incidence of postpartum haemorrhage, but has now become less common in some areas. An oxytocic drug is administered to expedite the third stage. Controlled cord traction is applied when the uterus contracts.

acupuncture Traditional Chinese therapy in which fine needles are inserted along specific lines or meridians in the body.

acupuncture point the point on the meridian at which the acupuncture needle is inserted.

acute describes a condition having a rapid onset, with pronounced symptoms but short duration.

acute abdomen name given to any condition which causes acute pain and tenderness over the abdomen.

acute circulatory failure inadequacy of the cardiovascular system to meet the tissue needs for gaseous, nutritive and other substances. May be due to loss of blood pressure from haemorrhage, loss of tension in the arteries or slow heartbeat.

acute inversion of the uterus a turning inside out of the uterus. A serious complication occurring when a medically-managed third stage of labour is mismanaged, such as when the uterus is not contracted before controlled cord traction is applied.

acute nephritis inflammation of the nephrons caused by infection, allergy or loss of blood supply. Characterized by proteinuria and haematuria.

acute renal failure a condition in which the kidneys are unable to secrete urine and maintain normal homeostasis due to inadequate blood flow or severe infection.

acute yellow atrophy of the liver (acute fatty liver disease) a rare complication seen in pregnancy, in which there is fatty necrosis, atrophy and destruction of the liver. Jaundice and itching will be the first symptoms.

adactylia congenital absence of fingers or toes.

adaptation the ability to adjust in structure, form or function.

addict a person who cannot function physically or emotionally without the aid of habitually used substances.

addiction a craving for, or loss of function without, the presence of the substance to which the body has become habituated.

additive a substance added to another to create a specific characteristic; a drug or chemical which may be added to another drug, intravenous infusion or food and administered at the same time.

adduction the movement of body parts towards each other or the mid-line of the body.

adherent placenta a placenta which has stuck fast to the myometrium and does not separate during the third stage of labour. It is unlikely to bleed and may be left in situ but may become infected. Surgical removal can be performed.

adhesion abnormal fibrous joining together of normally separate body parts or organs including parts of the intestines following caesarean section.

adipose tissue connective tissue containing fat cells and fibrous areolar bands.

ad lib (LATIN, *ad libitum*) give freely, to the desired amount.

admission the procedure or right of entry; process followed in registering a person for care in hospital.

adnexa adjoining or accessory organs or tissues; the uterine adnexa are the ovaries and fallopian tubes.

adnexal relating to adnexa.

adolescence the period between puberty and adulthood; the teenage years.

adoption a legal process by which the biological parent relinquishes parental responsibility for a child and non-biological parents acquire all rights and responsibilities.

adrenal glands two endocrine glands which are situated on the upper poles of the kidneys, the hormones of which regulate fluid and electrolyte balance, metabolic rate and the 'fight or flight' system.

adrenaline (US: epinephrine) one of the hormones secreted by the medulla of the adrenal gland.

adrenocorticotrophic hormone (ACTH) hormone secreted by the anterior pituitary and acting on the adrenal cortex.

adverse reaction severe, life-threatening response to the administration of e.g. a drug, the opposite or contrary effect not occurring in the majority of people receiving similar treatment.

advocacy to act or intercede on behalf of another and in the best interest of another person.

aer- prefix meaning air or oxygen gas.

aerobe an organism requiring oxygen for maintenance of life.

aerobic requiring air or free oxygen for metabolism and life.

aerobic exercise exercises done to increase the work of the heart and metabolism in order to maintain fitness.

aetiology the study of factors related to the causes and origins of disease (e.g. lifestyle, genetics, social conditions).

afferent carrying towards the centre – e.g. nerves towards the spinal column, blood vessels to the heart.

affiliation order a court order requiring a father to pay towards a child's support.

afibrinogenaemia loss of fibrin from the blood; occurs in association with disseminated intravascular coagulation (DIC), a complication of hypertension in pregnancy or catastrophic haemorrhage.

AFP *see* alphafetoprotein.

afterbirth the colloquial name given to the placenta and membranes expelled from the uterus after the birth of the baby.

aftercoming head the head following the birth of the body in a breech delivery.

afterpains painful contractions of the uterus occurring after delivery and commonly felt by multigravid women in the early puerperium and especially during breastfeeding.

agalactia a lack of breast milk.

age of consent 16 years; statutory age at which one may give permission for medical treatment and voluntary participation in sexual intercourse.

agenesis absence of an organ.

agenitalism a body without recognizable sex organs.

agglutination a process of clumping or coalescence.

agglutinin an antibody found in serum which, when added to an antigen on the surface of the erythrocyte results in agglutination of cells.

agglutinogen an antigen which when injected into the body stimulates the formation of agglutinin and causes agglutination.

agnathocephaly a congenital abnormality in which there is a small chin, displaced mouth and approximate fusion of the eyes, which are low set.

agranulocyte a leukocyte (white blood cell) which, unlike a monocyte or a lymphocyte, does not contain granules.

AID (artificial insemination by donor) becoming pregnant following injection into the uterus of semen from an anonymous man.

AIDS *see* acquired immune deficiency syndrome.

AIH (artificial insemination by husband) introduction of partner or husband's semen into the uterus by means not associated with sexual intercourse.

air the mixture of atmospheric gases surrounding the earth containing approximately 21% oxygen and 69% other gases and capable of sustaining respiration.

air embolism the abnormal presence of air in the vascular system or heart causing an obstruction to blood flow. Can be fatal.

air hunger a type of deep sighing respiration caused by imbalance of gases in the blood stimulating the respiratory centre.

air passages all the spaces through which air passes – nares, nasal cavity, pharynx, mouth, larynx, trachea and bronchial tree – on its way towards the lungs.

airborne infections transmission of pathogenic organisms on droplets of moisture in the air from one person to another without direct contact.

airway any of the devices used to maintain patency of the respiratory passages and prevent obstruction, used during anaesthesia and recovery.

ala wing-like processes or projection usually of bone, e.g. *ala of the sacrum.*

alba white substance, e.g. *lochia alba* (*see under* lochia).

albicans white, e.g. *Candida albicans.*

albinism hereditary condition in which there is a lack of the pigment melanin in the skin such that the skin, hair and eyes are devoid of colour. The condition may also be associated with visual problems.

albumin a protein substance which is the main constituent of animal tissues. Serum albumin found in the blood is essential for carrying bilirubin.

albuminuria the presence of albumin in the urine.

alcohol a fluid containing inflammable, intoxicating spirits which alters the cerebral function and consciousness. Consumption of alcohol in pregnancy should be restricted.

aldosterone hormone secreted by the adrenal cortex which has diuretic properties.

Alexander technique a method of psycho-physical training in relaxation which can help a woman cope with the demands of pregnancy and labour.

alignment organs or tissues are in optimal position to one another, e.g. when an episiotomy is repaired the edges must be in alignment to ensure future comfort and function.

alimentary pertaining to food or nutrition, as in *alimentary tract* – the whole digestive canal from mouth to anus.

alkalaemia a change in the pH level of the blood from 7.4 to a slightly alkaline pH which will be detrimental to health.

alkali a compound which reacts with acids to form salts.

alkalinity the quality of being alkaline, containing more hydroxyl than hydrogen ions. Fluids can be measured on the acid–base balance (pH) on a scale of 0 to 14, strong alkalines being 14 and strong acids 1. Water, being mid-scale and neutral, has a pH of 7 and blood a pH of 7.4.

alkaloids organic nitrogenous compounds, many of which are of medicinal value.

alkalosis an abnormal condition where the pH of body fluids is >pH 7.45 as a result of too much alkaline hydroxyl (bicarbonates) and not enough acid (hydrogen).

allergen a substance to which an individual has an abnormal response, such as itching skin, swelling, redness of the skin and mucous membranes including the eyelids.

allergic, allergy, allergic reaction a hypersensitivity reaction resulting from exposure to an allergen which may be a common substance in the environment such as pollen, feathers, etc. If the response is very severe, anaphylactic shock may occur, a condition which is life threatening.

alphafetoprotein (AFP) a by-product of fetal protein metabolism identifiable in maternal serum and amniotic fluid. Quantitative assessment can be used as the basis of an antenatal screening test for the detection of fetal abnormality, especially spina bifida, Down's syndrome and twin pregnancy. Further diagnostic tests are indicated.

alternative medicine a holistic approach to health and treatment not associated with Western medicine, e.g. homeopathy, massage, naturopathy or hypnosis. Women may use alternative medicine to relieve the discomfort of pregnancy, labour or the postnatal period as the side-effects which may occur with conventional Western medicine do not arise.

alveolus small hollow cavity (i.e. air pocket) in the lungs where oxygen is exchanged for carbon dioxide; the milk-secreting structures in the breasts.

amastia failure of development of secondary sex characteristics and congenital absence of breast tissue.

ambient surrounding, as in *ambient temperature*.

ambient temperature temperature of the surrounding air/environment. In a delivery suite the ambient air temperature will be above 25°C to prevent chilling the newborn.

amelia congenital absence of the extremity of one or more limbs.

amenorrhoea absence of the monthly menstrual bleed. While it may include the state of girls before menarche and women after the menopause, it is usually reserved for those of reproductive age and is a characteristic feature of pregnancy, certain diseases (e.g. anorexia nervosa) or severe emotional trauma.

amino acids a large group of organic compounds found in the blood; derived from protein in the diet and essential for building and repair of cells.

amitosis simple cell reproduction in which there is division of the nucleus and cytoplasm.

amnesia inability to remember experiences; loss of memory. May be due to trauma, emotions or artificially induced, so that the woman who is lightly anaesthetized during caesarean section does not recall the procedure.

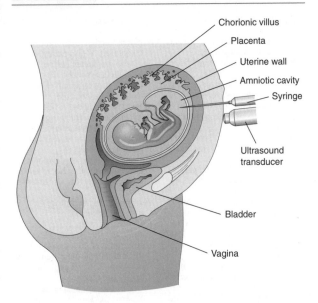

Chorionic villus
Placenta
Uterine wall
Amniotic cavity
Syringe
Ultrasound transducer
Bladder
Vagina

■ **Figure 4** Amniocentesis

amniocentesis an invasive procedure, performed around the 12th to 16th week of gestation, in which a large-bore needle is inserted through the abdominal wall and uterus into the amniotic sac and liquor amnii. Fluid containing fetal cells is withdrawn (*see* Figure 4). Fetal cells obtained are cultured for chromosomal abnormalities and karyotyping as one method of prenatal diagnosis. There is a risk of abortion occurring following this procedure.

amniohook an implement used to rupture the fetal membranes lining the uterus (*see* entry for amniotomy and Figure 7 below). Amniotic fluid drains and the pattern of labour may be changed.

amnioinfusion procedure to replace fluid which has drained off when membranes have ruptured prematurely and there is a risk of cord compression. Physiologically normal saline at body temperature is introduced into the amniotic cavity. Not currently routine practice in the UK.

amnion the inner of the two feto-placental membranes containing the amniotic fluid (liquor amnii) (*see* Figure 5).

amnionitis inflammation of the amniotic membrane due to infection.

amnioscopy introduction of a fibre optic instrument into the uterus to visualize the fetus.

amniotic cavity the space in the uterus occupied by the fetus, placenta, amniotic fluid, and lined by the amniotic membrane (*see* Figure 6).

amniotic fluid (SYNONYM liquor amnii) the almost colourless

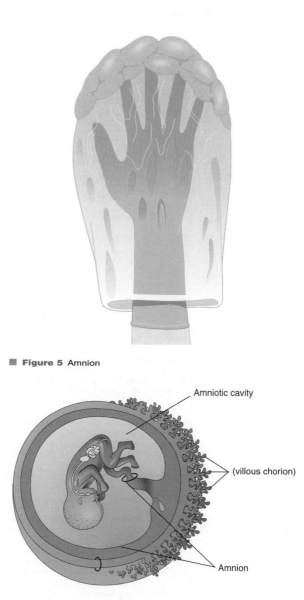

■ **Figure 5** Amnion

■ **Figure 6** Amniotic cavity

Amniotic cavity

(villous chorion)

Amnion

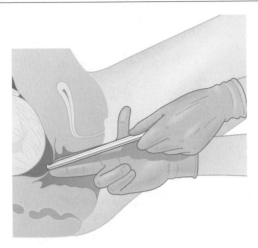

■ **Figure 7** Amniotomy

fluid surrounding the embryo and fetus in intrauterine life, thought to be formed by secretion from the amniotic membranes and fetal urine.

amniotic fluid embolism entry of liquor amnii into the maternal circulatory system. A rare and serious condition leading to shock and maternal collapse which can be fatal.

amniotic sac the membranes within which the fetus develops.

amniotomy the procedure of artificially rupturing the fetal or amniotic membranes (*see* Figure 7). Sometimes undertaken for observation of the liquor amnii as a means of assessment of the fetal condition, for the induction of labour, or to accelerate the first stage of labour. Carries risks; can increase pain and lead to further intervention.

ampulla the dilated end of a tube; the end of the fallopian tube furthest away from the uterus.

ampullary tubal pregnancy a conceptus which implants in the distal end of the fallopian tube rather than the uterus (*see* Figure 8).

anadidymus conjoined twins joined at the pelvis or lower.

anaemia lack of red blood cells, a low haemoglobin concentration or haematocrit on examination of the blood.

anaemia of pregnancy may be a true anaemia or may be a reduced haemoglobin due to haemodilution – termed physiological anaemia.

anaerobe a micro-organism not requiring oxygen to sustain growth.

anaerobic infection infection caused by organisms which do not need oxygen in order to multiply.

anaesthesia loss of consciousness induced by drugs prior to a painful surgical procedure such as caesarean section.

anaesthesia machine the apparatus used to maintain

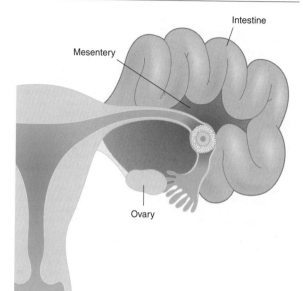

■ **Figure 8** Ampullary tubal pregnancy

the patient in an unconscious state by continuous administration of anaesthetic gases and artificial respiration.

anaesthetic agent used for inducing anaesthesia.

anaesthetist a doctor who specializes in care of the anaesthetized patient.

anal (COMBINING FORM ano-) pertaining to the anus, as in *anal incontinence, anoplasty.*

anal incontinence involuntary leakage of faeces due to defective functioning of the anal sphincter which closes the rectum.

anal orifice the opening into the rectum.

anal verge the margins or edges of the sphincter which closes the rectum. Can be damaged in childbirth.

analgesia an agent used to render a person or area of tissue insensitive to pain without loss of consciousness.

analgesic drug used to produce analgesia.

analysis the breakdown of fluids or concepts, including research, into their component parts.

anaphylactic reaction, anaphylactic shock a collapsed state induced by hypersensitivity to an antigen; the term applied to the respiratory distress and circulatory collapse that may be caused by snake venom, bee sting, a vaccine or certain foods.

anaphylaxis a severe allergic reaction. Soft tissues swell up and the airways can become obstructed making the condition fatal. An injection of adrenaline (epinephrine) is often given in an attempt to reverse this process.

anastomosis the creating of an opening between two cavities, tubes or organs. It may occur spontaneously or be accidentally or deliberately created during a surgical procedure.

anatomy the branch of science relating to the relationship between different tissues and organs of the body.

ancillary staff, ancillary services, ancillary support a person, service or support provided in addition to central activities, e.g. maternity care workers support the midwife and supplement the care she or he provides.

andro- prefix meaning man or masculine.

androgen a hormone believed responsible for promoting male secondary sex characteristics and function.

android pertaining to the male gender.

android pelvis description of the deeper more conical shape of pelvis seen in some women which can cause labour to be prolonged or sometimes obstructed.

androsterone an androgenic steroid found in male urine.

anecdotal information based on observation or an account from one person.

anencephalia congenital absence of the bones forming the vault of the skull together with the cerebral hemispheres and cerebellum.

anencephalus a fetus with signs of partial or complete anencephalia.

aneuploid having an uneven number of chromosomes.

angiogram an X-ray image of a blood vessel into which dye has been injected. May be performed postnatally if a deep vein thrombosis is suspected.

angioma a tumour composed of vessels – haemangioma (blood) or lymphangioma (lymphatic).

angiotensin a protein which causes vasoconstriction thereby raising the blood pressure. It is thought to be overactive in pregnancy-induced hypertension (PIH).

angle of inclination of the pelvis the angle formed by the horizontal plane of the pelvis with the anteroposterior diameter of the pelvic inlet.

ankyloglossia a congenital abnormality in which the frenulum of the tongue is shortened prohibiting movement and speech; tongue tie.

anococcygeal referring to the anus and coccyx, and the muscles between them.

anococcygeal body a mass of muscular and fibrous tissue situated between the anal canal and the coccyx.

anomaly a deviation from the normal.

anoplasty an operation performed to refashion the anus. Sometimes offered after a fourth degree tear.

anorchia the absence of one or both testicles.

anorexia nervosa an eating disorder of psychological origin characterized by aversion to food; predominantly affects teenagers and results in emaciation and amenorrhoea.

anorgasmy (anorgasmia) failure to experience orgasm.

anovular unassociated with ovulation.

anovular menstruation menstruation not associated with the prior release of an ovum.

anoxaemia low level of oxygen in the blood; associated with asphyxia.

anoxia a state without oxygen; asphyxia.

antacid a pharmacological preparation used for neutralizing acid in the stomach.

antagonist a drug that neutralizes or counteracts the effect of another.

antagonize to neutralize the effect of a substance.

ante- prefix denoting before or preceding.

anteflexion bending forward. Used to describe the position of the uterine fundus in relation to the cervix and vagina.

antenatal (SYNONYM prenatal) occurring before birth; during pregnancy.

antenatal care a series of observations of mother and fetus to detect and investigate risk factors and deviations from normal in the well-being of the mother and development of the fetus. Counselling and preparation for labour and childcare are included.

antenatal haemorrhage bleeding seen per vaginum during pregnancy; indicates a deviation from normal, e.g. placenta praevia, abruptio placentae, cervical infection or erosion.

antepartum before birth.

anterior situated before or to the front, referring to the forward part of an organ.

anterior fontanelle the fibromembranous area on the head of the fetus or neonate situated between the frontal, sagittal and coronal sutures.

anterior–posterior diameter of pelvic outlet the distance between the middle of the symphysis pubis and the upper edge of the third sacral vertebra. Should it be <10 cm there is a risk of cephalopelvic disproportion occurring in labour.

anteroposterior from front to back.

anteroposterior vaginal repair surgical procedure in which the upper and lower walls of the vagina are refashioned to reduce problems caused by overstretching and damage during the second stage of labour.

anteversion, anteverted inclined or tilted forward. The uterus is normally anteverted.

anthropoid ape-like, as in *anthropoid pelvis.*

anthropoid pelvis ape-like in character, the anteroposterior diameter is much greater than the transverse diameter. There is more space posteriorly than anteriorly so occipitoposterior positions of the fetus are more likely.

anthropology the study of people and their development, e.g. over time (*evolutionary anthropology*) and in relation to culture or rituals (*cultural anthropology*).

anti- prefix meaning against or preventing.

antibacterial preventing the growth of bacteria, usually a fluid or lotion.

antibiotic an antibacterial preparation or medicine offered when bacterial infection is present.

antibiotic resistance organisms not affected by antibiotics; symptoms of infection continue.

antibodies a class of substances formed by the body in response to an antigen.

antibody titre the strength or quantity of antibodies present. These are measured in a series and comparisons of the levels made; the level measured may indicate recent or past exposure to an antigen. If levels are rising this indicates that the body is currently fighting antigens or infection.

anticoagulant a substance which prevents or retards clot formation.

anticonvulsant a therapeutic agent that prevents or stops convulsions.

anti-D gamma globulin antirhesus antibody offered to rhesus negative women where there has been the probability of entry of fetal rhesus positive blood into the maternal circulation to prevent her forming her own antibodies. Fetal cells are coated with the globulin so the mother's body does not recognize them as a foreign protein. (*See* Appendix.)

antidepressants drugs used in the treatment of depression.

antidiuretic hormone the secretion of the adrenal gland which prevents excretion of urine, thereby controlling water loss from the body.

antidote an agent used to counteract the effect of poison or drug.

antiemetic drug given orally or by injection to prevent or treat nausea and vomiting.

antifungal a drug or cream which prevents growths of fungi. During pregnancy *Candida albicans* in the vagina is not uncommon; it may be treated with antifungal cream or pessaries.

antigalactic a drug which suppresses the formation of milk in the mammary glands.

antigen a substance that brings about production of antibodies as an immunologic response.

antihistamines a group of drugs used to block or diminish production of histamine which is released following tissue damage. Used in the treatment of various allergic conditions, e.g. hay fever.

antihypertensive a drug which lowers blood pressure.

antimicrobial a drug which prevents the growth of microscopic organisms.

antipruritic a drug, lotion or cream which is effective in the treatment of itching.

antipyretic a drug given to reduce a high body temperature

and alleviate the symptoms of fever.

antiseptic a lotion which discourages the growth of microorganisms.

antiseptic dressing a sterile pad or strips of gauze possibly impregnated with an antiseptic; used to cover a wound to prevent growth of or contamination by micro-organisms.

antiserum any serum obtained from human or animal blood which contains naturally derived antibody properties as a response to exposure to a specific disease. This can be injected into another person with the aim of protecting them from the disease, e.g. tetanus.

antispasmodic relieving or preventing spasm of smooth or striped (striated) muscle.

antithrombotic stocking applied to the legs to enhance the circulation thereby preventing the formation of clots. Routinely applied before caesarean section in some maternity units.

antitoxin an antibody prepared from blood or plasma of an infected person or animal and introduced into another to counteract the toxin causing damage to the body.

anuria no urine is being formed.

anus the terminal end of the digestive tract.

aorta the large arching artery arising from the left ventricle of the heart.

aortocaval compression inability of the vena cava to return blood to the heart and the aorta to pump it to the lower limbs due to restricted lumen caused by the weight of the pregnant uterus (*see* Figure 9). Occurs when the woman is lying on her back in the third trimester of pregnancy.

apareunia inability to perform sexual intercourse for

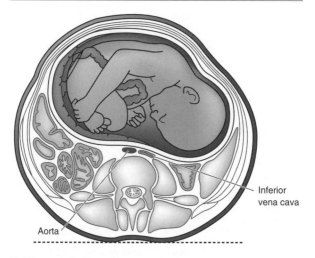

Inferior
vena cava

Aorta

■ Figure 9 Aortocaval compression

physiological or psychological reasons.

aperient laxative or purgative which will cause bowels to move, relieving constipation.

Apgar score a quantitative scoring mechanism used for determining the condition of the infant within 1, 5 and 10 minutes after birth and which may indicate the need for resuscitation. It assesses five features with a maximum score of 2 being assigned to each: heart rate; respiratory effort; muscle tone; response to stimuli; colour. (*See* Appendix.)

aplastic incomplete or defective structural development.

apnoea the absence or cessation of respiration; no breathing movement.

apnoea alarm mattress, apnoea monitor a machine which records breathing and sounds an alarm if breathing stops. A small pad on which a baby lies and which sounds an alarm if the baby stops breathing. Used for babies at risk of sudden infant death syndrome (SIDS).

applicator hollow rod used to introduce a soft structure (e.g. a tampon) or medicine (e.g. pessary) into a part of the body which cannot easily be reached.

appropriate for gestational age (AGA) a chart which compares the expected and attained growth of a fetus in utero at any stage of pregnancy.

approximate to situate next to each other; to bring two tissue surfaces together, as in the repair of a tear or episiotomy.

apyrexia no fever present.

aqua (LATIN) water.

aqua birth birth under water.

aquanatal exercises antenatal exercises, often in a local swimming pool, run by a trained midwife or other attendant to help mothers stay fit and develop social networks for postnatal support.

aqueous solution a water based fluid which may carry other substances dissolved in it.

arachnoid the web-like delicate middle meningeal membranes covering the brain and spinal cord.

arbor vitae uteri ridge-like folds of mucosa found within the uterine cervix.

arcing spring contraceptive device a diaphragm introduced into the vagina to act as a barrier to sperm penetration.

arcuate ligament the ligament stretching across the subpubic arch of the pelvis.

areola the coloured or pigmented area surrounding the nipple, which extends in pregnancy; usually, all of the areola needs to be in the baby's mouth for successful breast-feeding.

areolitis inflammation of the areola around the nipple as a result of cracked nipples and poor feeding position.

arm prolapse occurs when the cervix has dilated and the membranes rupture with the fetus in a transverse lie. The arm passes through the cervix and may be seen or felt protruding (*see* Figure 10). An emergency caesarean section may be required.

aromatic bath bath to which pleasant smelling oils or lotions have been added, used therapeutically to enhance mood and induce a feeling of well-being.

arrested development cessation of expected progress towards maturity.

arrested labour cessation in the progress of giving birth, possibly due to an obstruction.

arterial bleeding bleeding from an artery – identified by bright red blood and the pulsating nature of the flow.

arterial blood gas (ABG) the levels and pressures of oxygen

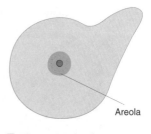

■ **Figure 10** Areola

and carbon dioxide in the blood of an artery. Measured in the blood of the umbilical artery in high risk cases where fetal hypoxia is suspected.

arterial line (A line) a catheter inserted into an artery to obtain a continuous reading of the arterial blood pressure; sometimes used following severe obstetric emergency involving maternal collapse.

arterial pH the measurement of the blood against the acid–alkaline balance.

arteriole small artery.

arteriosclerosis degenerative changes in the arteries resulting in thickening of the walls and making them less receptive to peristalsis.

artery a vessel carrying blood away from the heart.

artery forceps an instrument with locked scissor-like handles and flat serrated blades; used to clamp a bleeding vessel or hold tissue during surgical procedures.

arthritis inflammation of joints.

articulate unification of one or more joints; movement of one or more joints together.

articulation of the pelvis the relationship in degrees between the plane of the pelvis with the horizontal plane and the spine.

artificial feeding the maintenance of feeding by means other than the mouth. When used in relation to the infant it refers to the giving of food other than mother's milk by mouth; usually in a bottle or via a tube or cup.

artificial insemination introduction of sperm into the uterus by mechanical means rather than by sexual intercourse to achieve fertilization and pregnancy. *Artificial insemination by donor* (AID) – using sperm from a donor so one biological parent will be unknown. *Artificial insemination by husband* (AIH) – using sperm from the woman's partner or husband.

artificial respiration the maintenance of breathing by mouth to mouth (or mouth to mouth and nose) from another person or by a machine.

artificial rupture of membranes (ARM) the amniotic membranes are punctured and amniotic fluid released; often carried out to speed up labour and to see if meconium has been passed indicating fetal distress. Side-effects include increased pain, increased likelihood of further intervention in labour and, occasionally, cord prolapse.

ascites collection of free fluid in the peritoneal cavity; usually associated with heart failure. When seen in the fetus it is associated with severe anaemia and hydrops fetalis.

asepsis the complete absence of microscopic organisms or bacteria.

aseptic technique a procedure undertaken using sterile equipment and technique so that micro-organisms will not be introduced into the body.

asexual without reference to gender; without sex organs.

asoma a fetus without a complete trunk and head.

aspermia failure of spermatozoa to mature.

aspermatogenesis testicles do not produce sperm.

asphyxia oxygen deprivation. *Asphyxia neonatorum* is failure of initiation of respiration in the newborn infant. Blood oxygen levels are low and the carbon dioxide level is very high.

aspiration the process of drawing up of fluid or gases from a cavity by suction. Meconium aspiration occurs when meconium has been passed before birth and entered the lungs in utero or during the first few breaths after birth.

aspiration pneumonia pneumonia caused by inhalation of infected materials from the upper respiratory tract or gastric content; burning of the lung lining by acid drawn up from the stomach and then inhaled.

aspirator an implement used to which negative pressure is applied to draw fluid or gas from a cavity.

assertiveness the ability to communicate one's opinions and rights effectively without being overbearing and without denying those of other people.

assertiveness training programme or course designed to help midwives understand the need to communicate effectively and confidently so they can become the woman's advocate during her time of vulnerability.

assessing collecting information regarding situation, history, progress or behaviour and comparing it to set of criteria in order to establish risk or achievement.

assessment a statement of evaluation or appraisal of behaviour or progress towards a goal.

assisted breech medical approach to delivering the fetus presenting by the breech vaginally; assistance is given by applying forceps to the head to achieve a controlled delivery.

assisted reproductive technology the branch of medicine which helps infertile couples to conceive a baby.

Association for Improvements in the Maternity Services (AIMS) a charitable organization led by non-professional women who support childbearing women in ensuring that their needs are met by the maternity services and who lobby for political change. AIMS also produces literature informing women about their choices in different areas.

Association of Radical Midwives an organization originally set up by student midwives who felt that changes were needed in midwifery practice. The term 'radical' relates to a desire to return to the roots of practice rather than indicating a particular political position. Members lobby for political change, woman-centred care and autonomous midwifery practice.

asthma a respiratory condition in which there is muscle spasm causing narrowing of the trachea and bronchi, thus creating difficulties in breathing with accompanying cough and wheezing sound on expiration. Asthma usually improves for the duration of a pregnancy.

asymmetric two halves or parts of the same, which should look and behave the same but do not.

asymmetry lack of balance between two similar structures. One side is not the same as the other.

asynclitism the position of the baby's head within the pelvis where one of the parietal bones is further down than the other. Usually, the baby's head needs to move to a synclitic position in order to negotiate the pelvis.

This can be achieved in practice by encouraging maternal asymmetrical positions.

at risk term describing a client in whom there is a greater than normal likelihood of an abnormality or life-threatening condition arising.

atelectasis incomplete inflation of the lungs. This may be primary failure at birth or secondary to obstruction and collapse. Seen especially in preterm babies.

atlas the first cervical vertebra, which moves under the occipital bone.

atony absence of muscle tone.

atresia blind end or closure of a normally open canal. In the neonate it can be associated with the oesophagus or anus as a congenital abnormality.

atrial septal defect a congenital condition in which the septum of the heart is abnormal – usually there is a hole allowing communication between the left and right atria (*see* Figure 11).

atrium the singular name for the upper chambers of the heart (PLURAL atria).

atrophic vaginitis degeneration of the vaginal mucous membrane, usually after the menopause, leading to a reduction in size.

atrophy withered degeneration of cells leading to a reduction in their size.

atropine (hyoscyamine) An alkaloid extract of the belladonna plant (*Atropa belladonna*) administered prior to surgery for reducing secretions of the gastrointestinal and respiratory tracts and to induce muscle relaxation.

attachment being fixed to another structure for stability; dependent emotionally on another individual, as in the baby's attachment to the mother.

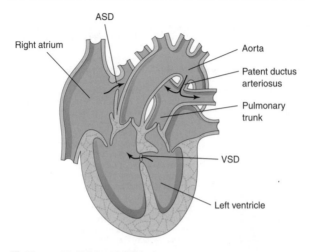

ASD
Right atrium
Aorta
Patent ductus arteriosus
Pulmonary trunk
VSD
Left ventricle

■ **Figure 11** Atrial septal defect

attachment parenting an approach to parenting where the baby is kept close to the mother and/or another person in order to help promote feelings of security. Usually includes breastfeeding and co-sleeping.

attitude relating to position or posture. The relationship of the fetal parts to each other, e.g. head to spine.

atypical differing from what might normally be expected.

audio- combining form meaning associated with the sense of hearing. *Auditory* has the same meaning.

audit a means of evaluating care and its relationship to research and expected standards. Changes can be made as a result to enable expected standards to be achieved.

augment to accelerate or intensify an established process, as in the use of oxytocin in a labour that is slow to progress.

augmentation a procedure in which a substance is given to stimulate or accelerate a normal physiological process.

aura a warning sensation experienced by a person with epilepsy before a fit.

aural relating to the ear.

auscultation the process of listening to the sounds emitted by internal organs; listening to the fetal heartbeat in pregnancy.

authentic the quality of being open and honest in behaviour and motives; genuine or original.

autohypnosis the ability to induce a trance in oneself, and to become unaware of the world around. Some women use self-hypnosis to enable them to cope with the pain of labour.

autolysis (self-ingestion) the spontaneous breakdown of body tissues by enzymes. The uterine size is reduced to a non-pregnant size by this process 6 weeks after birth.

autonomic involuntary or independent of one's will or control, as, for example, the functioning of the *autonomic nervous system.*

autonomic nervous system the part of the nervous system which regulates smooth or involuntary muscles. The sympathetic nerves speed up contractions and gland secretion and increase muscle tone. The parasympathetic nerves reverse these processes.

autonomy right of self-government; the ability of the midwife to practise on her own responsibility for women in normal pregnancy and childbirth.

autopsy (SYNONYM postmortem) examination after death to determine the cause or improve understanding of disease progression.

autosomal dominant inheritance the gene carrying markers for a specific disease will cause that condition in the presence of a healthy paired partner.

autosomal recessive inheritance two affected genes need to have been inherited for the medical condition to be manifested, e.g. phenylketonuria.

autosome a chromosome that is non-sex determined.

autozygous genes which are copies of ancestral genes and the result of a consanguineous union.

average a value which is representative of a series of numbers or items. The *mean average* is calculated by adding the sum of a series of numbers and dividing it by the number of items in the series; the *mode* (most frequently occurring number or item) and the *median* (central number when all are placed in order) *averages* may also be used.

axilla (SYNONYM armpit) the hollow depression beneath the arm and chest.

axillary pertaining to the axilla.

axillary node a lymph gland found in the armpit.

axillary tail of Spence breast tissue found under the armpit.

axillary temperature the body temperature recorded by placing a thermometer under the armpit for 3 minutes.

axis an imaginary line passing through the centre of the body; the second cervical vertebra, over which the atlas moves.

axis traction the process of pulling on the fetal head to aid delivery when progress in the second stage of labour is arrested.

Bb

B one of the antigens found on red cells, present in human blood groups B and AB.

Babinski's reflex an abnormal reflex in which the great toe extends and the other toes fan out when the lateral aspect of the foot is stroked.

baby bottle tooth decay premature tooth decay caused by long exposure to milk or juice when the infant is allowed to sleep while sucking a bottle.

Baby Friendly Initiative a campaign initiated by UNICEF to encourage all mothers to breastfeed thereby giving all children the associated advantages. Maternity units are offered a status incentive to work towards improving breastfeeding rates.

bacillary rod-shaped; relating to a bacillus.

bacille Calmette-Guérin (BCG) an attenuated (weakened) strain of tubercle bacillus used in vaccines to immunize against tuberculosis.

bacillus (PLURAL bacilli) a generic term for any rod-like bacterial organism; a bacterium of the genus *Bacillus* (family Bacillaceae).

backache pain located over the lumbar region of the back; occurs frequently in pregnancy due to changes in the centre of gravity as the uterus becomes heavier.

bacteraemia presence of bacteria in the blood.

bacteria (SINGULAR bacterium) a group of single-celled microscopic organisms universally found in plants and animals.

Some of these can be disease-forming when they enter the body. Others can be protective.

bacterial shock a state of shock with severe hypotension and circulatory failure resulting from bacteraemia.

bactericide an agent that destroys bacteria.

bacteriology the scientific study of bacteria.

bacteriostatic an agent capable of arresting bacterial growth.

bacteriuria presence of bacteria in the urine.

bag of waters common name for the liquor contained in the amniotic membranes.

balanic refers to the glans penis in the male and the clitoris in the female.

balanitis inflammation of the glans penis. In babies it may indicate the need for more frequent changes of nappy.

ballottement a diagnostic procedure used to determine the presence of a floating organ or object such as a fetus. The object or organ is pushed or tapped to encourage displacement and rebound of content against the containing wall such that the impact is palpable (*see* Figure 12).

Bandl's ring the pathological thickening of the normal retraction ring that occurs when labour is obstructed. If it is palpable abdominally it is an indication of imminent uterine rupture.

bar graph an easily-interpreted method of presenting data so that the total distribution of

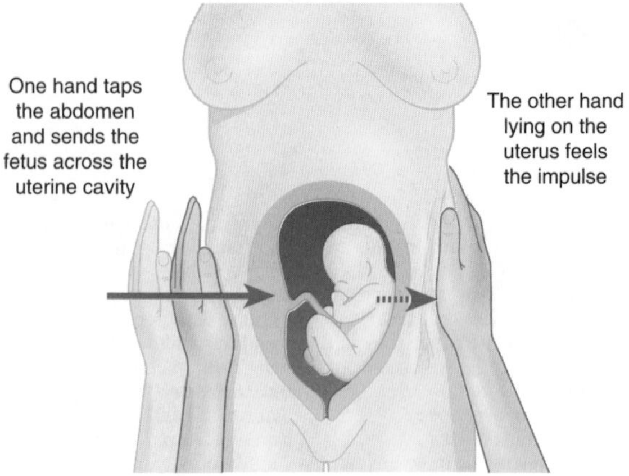

One hand taps the abdomen and sends the fetus across the uterine cavity

The other hand lying on the uterus feels the impulse

■ **Figure 12** Ballottement

outcomes may be seen at one time in proportion to each other.

barbiturates a group of drugs acting on the brain to produce a hypnotic and sedative effect.

Barlow's test a test done to diagnose congenital dislocation of the hips.

barrier nursing nursing care carried out when a patient is in isolation to prevent the spread of infection.

Bartholinitis inflammation of a Bartholin's gland. Can result in cystic or abscess formation.

Bartholin's glands glands situated on either side of the lower part of the vagina, the secretions of which lubricate the vagina.

Bart's test a blood test offered at 16–18 weeks' gestation to identify women at high risk of having an abnormal fetus. Now more commonly known as the *double, triple* or *quadruple test.* (*See* Appendix.)

basal metabolic rate a measure of the units of energy and oxygen used for production of heat by the body at rest. It is expressed as percentage above or below that used by others of the same height, weight and age. In pregnancy the basal metabolic rate is increased by up to 30%.

basal temperature the body's temperature is taken after rest and before rising. A rise of 0.5°C above the normal body temperature at the same time indicates that ovulation is imminent; the temperature will remain increased until the next menstrual period. Used as a means of natural family planning, sometimes in combination with other methods.

base the main component of a mixture; the bottom, e.g. the inferior aspect of the skull.

baseline fetal heart rate the fetal heart rate as measured in early labour, to which later patterns can be compared and

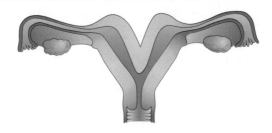

Figure 13 Bicornuate uterus

used for diagnosis of possible abnormalities.

basophil a leukocyte with an affinity for basic dyes making them easier to examine.

battledore placenta a placenta in which there is displacement of the umbilical cord from the centre to the side.

BCG *see* bacille Calmette-Guérin.

b.d. (LATIN, *bis die*) twice daily. Used in prescribing to indicate how often to give medicine.

bearing down describes both the sensation and action of the expulsive contractions experienced during the second stage of labour, where the woman pushes, involuntarily or with added effort, in order to move her baby through the birth canal.

bed rest curtailment of all ambulatory activities and restriction to rest in bed as a means of preserving a threatened abortion. Its effectiveness is not scientifically proven.

Bell's palsy paralysis of the face caused by facial nerve damage; this may be as a result of trauma during a forceps delivery, shoulder dystocia, exposure to cold or viral infection.

Benedict's test a qualitative reaction test used for identification of glucose and other reducing substances in urine.

benign non-malignant; not dangerous to life.

beta (β) denoting second. Often combined with the name of another substance or compound.

beta-haemolytic streptococcus a streptococcal bacterium that is potentially pathogenic and can be fatal to the neonate.

betamethasone a steroid. Sometimes offered to women in preterm labour as it increases the level of lecithin in the fetal lungs helping to maintain expansion and reducing the risk of respiratory distress syndrome (RDS) after birth.

bi-, bin- prefix, denoting two.

biased sample a selective group of individuals used in research who are likely to be of similar opinion; the research result will therefore be subjective rather than objective and some validity may be lost.

bicarbonate a salt of carbonic acid. Sodium bicarbonate is used to correct acidaemia.

bicornuate uterus congenital abnormality in which there is incomplete fusion of the two tubes which unite to form the uterus. The uterus is heart-shaped or has a septum (bicornuate or bicornate, having two horns; *see* Figure 13). Contractions are less efficient and placental retention is common.

bidet a large basin with pedestal on which one can sit to wash the genital and rectal areas.

bigeminal pregnancy a twin pregnancy.

bilateral referring to both sides of the body.

bile a bitter greenish alkaline substance secreted by the liver whose function is to aid breakdown and absorption of fats in the intestines.

bilirubin a product resulting from the breakdown of haemoglobin. It is the main pigment found in bile. It is insoluble in water, but once conjugated by the liver it can be excreted in faeces and urine. In neonatal life the liver is immature and haemolysis is excessive. The bilirubin will remain fat-soluble and be stored in the skin which will subsequently appear yellow (jaundiced).

bilirubinaemia high levels of red/orange bile pigment circulating in the blood. Very high levels will stain fat yellow in the brain and may cause permanent damage (kernicterus).

bilirubinometer an instrument for measuring the concentration of bilirubin in blood.

Billing's method a means of determining the fertile period in the menstrual cycle by examination of the consistency of cervical mucus; the mucus becomes stretchy around the time of ovulation.

bilobate placenta a placenta having two large sections (lobes).

bimanual using both hands, as in *bimanual palpation,* an examination performed using two hands.

bimanual compression of the uterus a method used to arrest severe postpartum haemorrhage by squeezing the uterus. One hand is externally placed abdominally over the uterine fundus and the other formed into a fist within the vagina. The clinician compresses the uterus between the two hands (*see* Figure 14).

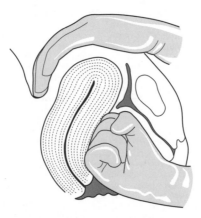

■ **Figure 14** Bimanual compression of uterus

bimanual palpation of the pelvic organs examination of the pelvic organs with one hand over the lower abdomen and two fingers of the other hand in the vagina (*see* Figure 15). Used for early pregnancy detection.

binovular derived from two separate ova, as in *binovular twin pregnancy.*

biochemistry the study of the chemicals, elements and their reactions within living tissues.

biological profile an estimate of fetal well-being using ultrasound to measure fetal heart rate, muscle tone, movements, breathing and amniotic fluid volume.

biology the scientific study of life, including botany and zoology.

biopsy the excision of tissue from a living body and its use for diagnostic study.

biparietal diameter measured distance between the parietal eminences of the fetal skull, made by the use of ultrasound scan. Used to estimate fetal growth and maturity and traditionally taken as 9.5 cm at term.

biparous a woman who has given birth to two infants in different pregnancies.

bipartite having two parts; a placenta can be called bipartite if there are two parts, not necessarily of equal size.

bipolar having two poles. A term commonly applied to the pregnant uterus.

birth asphyxia failure of the baby to breathe at birth.

birth canal a collective description of the birth passage which includes the soft and bony structures traversed by the fetus during vaginal birth.

birth centre a place where women can give birth in a homely atmosphere without medical intervention. It is staffed by midwives who can deal with emergencies when these occasionally arise, yet is not technologically equipped to deal with anticipated obstetric complications so is mainly an option for 'low-risk' women.

birth certificate a legal document recording details of a person's date and place of birth, gender, given name, names of

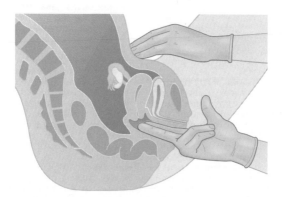

■ **Figure 15** Bimanual palpation of the pelvic organs

parents; used as a form of identification.

birth control methods used in the regulation and avoidance of conception.

birth injury damage such as intracranial haemorrhage, and brachial plexus nerve damage sustained by the fetus during birth.

birth mother the woman who gives birth to the baby, but not necessarily the genetic mother.

birth notification the requirement to give information of a birth to the district medical officer within 36 hours of the birth having taken place. The responsibility falls to any person present at the birth or attending within 6 hours, in practice usually the attending midwife.

birth plan a description by the mother of care she would like in labour.

birth rate the number of births per year per 100 of the mid-year population of women between the ages of 15 and 45 years.

birth registration the legal requirement that all births be registered in the district in which they have occurred within 42 days. Following registration, birth certification is issued, child benefits may be paid, and statistics required for local town planning will be collected.

birth trauma injury occurring during delivery; may be mild or severe, and injuries may be temporary or permanent.

birth weight weight of the baby immediately after birth. It is the baseline for assessing future weight gain, but it can be inaccurate, according to whether meconium has been passed or not and the cord milked or not. The UK national average is 3.5 kg but this figure has not

been reviewed for a number of years.

birthing chair chair designed to give the advantages of the upright position for the second stage of labour.

birthing stool crescent shaped stool on which a woman may sit for support during labour and birth.

birthmark a skin blemish present at birth; it may be either a pigmented naevus or a vascular haemangioma.

bisacromial diameter a measurement of the distance between the acromion processes of the shoulder blades. In the term fetus the bisacromial diameter measures approximately 12 cm.

bisexual possessing both male and female characteristics; in adults, a person who is sexually attracted to both women and men.

Bishop's score a method of assessing the condition of the cervix and its favourability for induction of labour. An unfavourable cervix may be ripened by the administration of prostaglandin gel or pessaries prior to induction. (*See* Appendix.)

bitemporal diameter measurement of the diameter between the coronal sutures taken at the inferior end, usually 8.2 cm at term.

bitrochanteric diameter the measured distance between the greater trochanters of the femur taken just below the neck. It is the engaging diameter when the fetus presents by the breech and is usually 10 cm at term.

bladder the hollow muscular sac that is a reservoir for urine before voiding.

blastocyst the primitive and early differentiation of the conceptus. It consists of trophoblast, inner cell mass and blastocele.

blastula an early stage in the development of a zygote as it progresses to become an embryo.

blastulation the transformation of the morula into a blastocyst.

bleed to lose blood from the circulation.

bleeding time the time taken to stop bleeding – 6 minutes in the non-pregnant state.

blighted ovum an abnormal ovum which grows, but not into an embryo.

block an obstruction. *Epidural block* occurs when the passage of impulses up the spinal cord has been stopped by local anaesthetic in the epidural space.

blood bank a refrigerated storage facility where blood for future transfusion is kept.

blood cell can be *red blood cells* (erythrocytes) or *white blood cells* (leukocytes).

blood clot a semi-solid or gelatinous mass resulting from the clumping together of various components in the blood to arrest a bleed.

blood cross-matching a test to assess compatibility of blood before transfusion. Recipient serum is mixed with donor cells or donor serum with recipient cells. If agglutination does not occur the blood is deemed compatible.

blood gases the concentration of oxygen, carbon dioxide and bicarbonate in the blood. Measured in fetal or cord blood in the delivery suite in neonates at risk of having suffered occult asphyxia.

blood group genetically determined classification of human erythrocytes based on the presence of specific antigens (agglutinogens) in the erythrocyte and antibodies (agglutinins) in the serum. Erythrocytes may also contain the rhesus antigen.

People whose red cells contain antigen are classified as rhesus positive (Rh+) and those without the antigen as rhesus negative (Rh−).

blood pH a measure of the acidity or alkalinity of blood. The average adult blood pH is 7.4.

blood pressure (BP) The pressure exerted by the blood on the vessel wall. When being measured as a screening or diagnostic procedure two measurements are taken. The first measurement, or systolic, is the maximum pressure within the brachial artery during contraction of the ventricles and the second, diastolic, the pressure within the artery when the ventricles are at rest.

blood sugar the amount of sugar (usually glucose) in the blood. The quantity varies and may rise following a meal and fall during fasting. The normal range in a healthy adult is between 3.3 and 5.3 mmol/L.

blood transfusion the taking of blood from one individual and administering it to another.

blood urea the quantity of urea in the blood – usually 2–6 mmol/dl.

blue baby a baby who remains centrally cyanosed after establishment of respiration at birth. Cyanosis may be due to a severe cardiac or pulmonary abnormality.

body image the conscious or unconscious perception a person has of their body. This may change in pregnancy, depending on the woman's attitude to being pregnant, and may be reflected in her behaviour and her feelings about herself.

body mass index (BMI) the relationship of weight to height expressed numerically. It indicates the amount of body fat and it is known that women with a high BMI do less well in labour. BMI < 20 = underweight. BMI > 30 = overweight.

body temperature heat produced by the body as a result of fuel metabolism. It is essential to maintain a stable environment for optimal functioning – usually between 36 and 37°C. In pregnancy the basal temperature may rise and the woman may feel warmer than people around her.

bonding the emotional attachment and dependence between a mother and her baby/child. Initiated at birth, bonding can be interrupted where mother and baby are unnecessarily separated, or where medical or midwifery procedures are carried out which disturb mother-baby contact.

booking the initial meeting between the midwife and pregnant woman, ideally before 12 weeks' gestation, when the woman's medical, family and obstetric history is recorded, needs for care are assessed, plans for care are drawn up, health counselling given and a relationship of trust established.

bottle feeding nourishment given to a baby by means of a bottle topped with a teat which is sucked. The bottle may contain modified cows' milk or expressed breast milk.

Bowman's capsule the glomerular capsule receiving the filtrate from the blood at the far end of the nephron in the kidney. It passes through the tubules where some reabsorption occurs.

brachial referring to the arm.

brachial artery an artery originating in the axilla that is palpable as it runs near the surface and anterior to the elbow, it branching at the elbow to supply the radius and ulna.

brachial plexus nerves just above the clavicle which can become overstretched during a breech or vaginal delivery resulting in Erb's paralysis or Klumpke's paralysis.

brachycephaly a congenital abnormality in which the coronal sutures on the skull close early in development and the head expands sideways in order for the brain to develop.

bradycardia an abnormally slow heart rate – below 60 beats per minute in an adult, or below 90 beats per minute in a fetus.

brain the main part of the central nervous system contained within the cranium and consisting of the cerebellum, cerebrum, pons and medulla oblongata.

Brandt–Andrews manoeuvre for delivering the placenta and membranes after separation. One hand holds the uterus while the other puts traction on the cord (*see* Figure 16). Should not be carried out during physiological third stage.

Braxton-Hicks contractions painless, intermittent contractions of the uterus occurring in pregnancy from 20 weeks' gestation.

breakthrough bleeding loss of blood from the uterus not associated with menstruation.

breast one of the two mammary glands situated on the anterior chest wall.

breast abscess infection and pus formation during lactation or weaning.

breast milk the nutritious substance secreted by the mammary glands; it appears 3–5 days after parturition and following the secretion of colostrum.

breast milk jaundice jaundice which starts in the first few weeks of life as a result of a substance (metabolite) in the

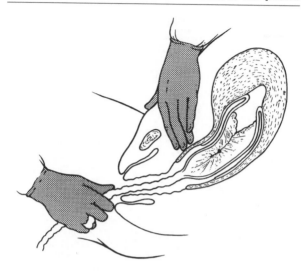

■ **Figure 16** Brandt–Andrews manoeuvre

mother's milk that inhibits the infant from conjugating bilirubin to a glucuronide which can be excreted. The jaundice is mild and may correct itself or remain for the duration of breastfeeding. It is not a contra-indication to breastfeeding.

breast pump apparatus for suctioning milk from the breast using hand or electric pumping action.

breastfeeding nourishing a baby by feeding milk from the breast(s).

breech the buttocks; the position when the fetus lies with its buttocks occupying the lower pole of the uterus (*see* Figure 17). Debate exists around whether breech presentation is a variation of the normal, or an abnormal occurrence where all women experiencing this should be offered routine external cephalic version or caesarean section.

breech extraction the medical assistance which may be provided at the delivery of an infant being born vaginally. The accoucheur may exert traction on the body or apply forceps to the aftercoming head. (*See also* physiological breech birth.)

breech presentation the fetus lies in the uterus with its buttocks or feet presenting first.

bregma the anterior fontanelle. The larger of the two fibromembranous regions on the fetal skull found at the junction of the frontal, coronal and sagittal sutures.

brim of the pelvis the circumscribed inlet to the bony part of the birth canal.

A Complete or full breech

B Frank breech

C Footling or incomplete breech

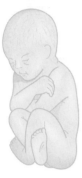
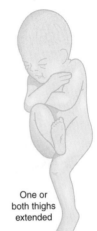

Fully flexed fetus

Not fully flexed fetus with legs extended

One or both thighs extended

■ **Figure 17** Breech

British Medical Association (BMA) a national professional organization for support of doctors.

British Pharmacopoeia (BP) a document stating the contents and preparation of medicines so that uniformity of prescription is achieved.

broad ligaments a double fold of peritoneum extending laterally from the uterus to the pelvic wall and enclosing the fallopian tubes (*see* Figure 18).

bromocriptine a drug used to inhibit prolactin secretion and thereby suppress lactation.

bronchopneumonia infection in the lungs with exudates settling in the bronchi and alveoli. May result from inhalation of meconium at birth.

bronchopulmonary dysplasia granular damage to the lungs associated with administration of high quantities of oxygen therapy in neonates with respiratory distress syndrome.

bronchus one of the primary branches of the trachea.

brow the upper anterior part of the head; forehead.

brow presentation when the fetus is a cephalic presentation, but the head is neither fully flexed nor fully extended (*see* Figure 19). The mento-vertical diameter, which at 13.5 cm is larger than any of the pelvic diameters, presents, which can lead to an obstruction of labour and cephalopelvic disproportion.

brown fat a type of adipose tissue, a particularly easily accessible energy store. Only

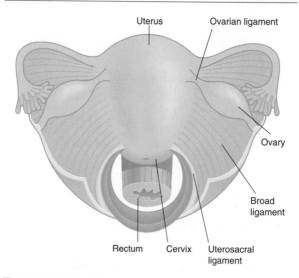

Figure 18 Broad ligament

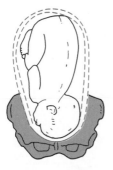

Figure 19 Brow presentation

found in the fetus and neonate, between the shoulder blades, neck, around the sternum and kidneys.

buccal referring to the cheek; some drugs may be adminis-tered into the *buccal pouch* (*see* Figure 20) from where they are easily absorbed across the mucous membrane into the bloodstream.

bulbocavernosus muscles of the pelvic floor which encircle the vaginal orifice.

bupivacaine (Marcain®) a local anaesthetic drug used for paracervical analgesic block or epidurals.

Burns–Marshall technique an older method of delivering the aftercoming head in a breech presentation. The ankles were held and slight traction exerted as the feet were carried through a wide arc up to and over the mother's abdomen. Has been shown to be potentially haz-ardous and should no longer be used.

buttonholing a term applied to the appearance of the perineum

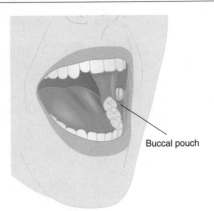

Buccal pouch

■ **Figure 20** Buccal pouch

as it is distended by the fetal head in the second stage of labour. The skin starts to tear along and within the perineal body indicating that a moderate to severe laceration will occur.

Cc

C symbolic representation for carbon.

C, c symbol used to denote rhesus blood types, others being D, d and E, e.

caesarean section surgical incision into the abdominal and uterine wall to achieve delivery of the baby (*see* Figure 21). It is done when continuation of the pregnancy or/and vaginal delivery would be hazardous for the mother or fetus. In a *lower segment caesarean section* (LSCS) the incision is made into the lower abdomen and the lower section of the uterus. A 'bikini-line' scar results.

caked breast a state of extreme engorgement of the breasts in which they become hard as the milk comes in and is not removed.

calamine a pink, odourless lotion based on zinc oxide and ferric oxide; applied to the skin to relieve itching.

calcaneum (SYNONYM calcaneus) the heel bone.

calcaneus valgus a type of talipes in which the ankle is flexed

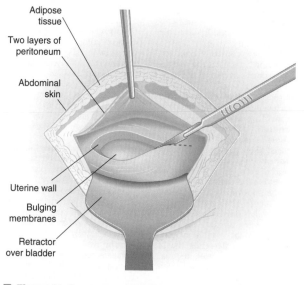

■ **Figure 21** Caesarean section layers

and only the heel touches the ground.

calcification deposition of calcium salt within body tissues; calcification of the mature placenta. The degree of calcification of the fetal bones is used to denote maturity.

calcium a metal with a strong affinity for oxygen; widely found in nature.

calcium phosphate one of three calcium salts. Essential to the formation of strong bones and teeth.

calculus (stone) a solid collection of mineral substances; may be found in the kidneys or gall bladder and requires surgical removal if symptoms of obstruction occur.

Caldwell–Moloy pelvic classification a system used for classifying the female pelvis as one of four types: gynaecoid, android, anthropoid and platypelloid.

callipers curved, hinged compasses for measuring diameter of convex bodies, for example the fetal skull.

callus new growth of bone tissue which forms at the margin of fractures as part of the healing process.

calorie a unit of heat or amount of fuel need to raise the temperature of 1 g of water by 1°C.

candida (*Candida albicans, Monilia albicans*) a fungus or yeast-like pathogen causing thrush.

candidiasis fungal infection found in the vagina, mouth and sometimes on the skin around the nipple. The neonate can be infected during breastfeeding.

canker sore an ulcer-like lesion on the genitals or in the mouth.

cannabis the flowering top of the hemp plant used to treat glaucoma and nausea and which can create an altered state of consciousness.

cannula an artificial tube inserted into the body cavity for delivery of drugs, fluids or to enable drainage of fluids. It is often fitted with a trocar for insertion.

cannulation the insertion of a cannula (narrow patent tube) into the body (*see* Figure 22). Midwives cannulate women's veins to administer fluids or drugs.

cap contraceptive diaphragm which covers the cervix to prevent entry of sperm; often used with a spermicide.

capillary minute, hair-like vessels connecting arteries, veins or the lymphatic system.

capillary haemangioma a birthmark on the skin made of tiny blood vessels.

caput succedaneum oedematous swelling on the presenting part of the head, occurring during labour when venous return is restricted by tight application of the cervix (*see* Figure 23).

carbohydrates a group of organic compounds which on ingestion by the body can be metabolized for energy, growth and repair of tissue.

carbon dioxide (CO_2) an odourless, colourless gas present in small quantities in the atmosphere. It is also a by-product of tissue oxidation and is excreted via the lungs.

carbon dioxide tension the partial pressure of carbon dioxide gas in the blood. Its measurement usually reflects pulmonary gaseous exchange. The quality present in blood obtained from the fetus or umbilical cord can indicate the degree of asphyxia or otherwise.

carbon monoxide a highly toxic gas produced by combustion. It has a high affinity with haemoglobin to which it binds, preventing uptake of oxygen.

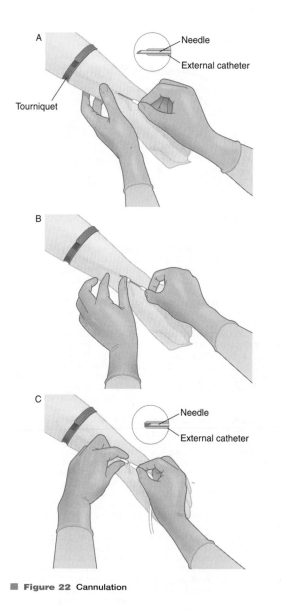

Figure 22 Cannulation

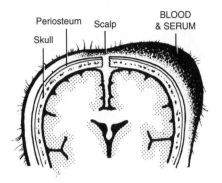

Skull · Periosteum · Scalp · BLOOD & SERUM

■ **Figure 23** Caput succedaneum

Present in the bodies of people who smoke cigarettes and those who passively inhale cigarette smoke.

carboxyhaemoglobin the displacement of oxygen from erythrocyte and replacement with carbon dioxide.

carcinogen an agent which may cause a carcinoma to develop.

carcinoma a malignant tumour or uncontrolled growth of cells structurally and functionally different from and disruptive to those around them.

cardiac arrest cessation of heart contractions and failure of cardiac output. In labouring women this may be due to drug reaction, severe haemorrhage or other obstetric emergency. (*See* Appendix.)

cardiac massage rhythmic repeated downward pressure on the sternum to compress the heart and so maintain circulation.

cardiac output the amount of blood (expressed in litres) ejected by the left ventricle of the heart in 1 minute. Normal values are increased in pregnancy due to increased blood volume.

cardiac sphincter the round muscle between the stomach and the oesophagus. In pregnancy the muscle may be slightly relaxed allowing reflux of gastric juices into the oesophagus or mouth causing heartburn.

cardinal ligament (SYNONYM transverse cervical ligament) the lower thickened portions of the broad ligament which is firmly anchored to the cervix and lateral walls of the pelvis, providing support to the uterus.

cardinal movements of labour the principal positions and movements of the fetus during its passage through the birth canal.

cardiography an electronic recorded trace of heart movement and function.

cardiotocography (CTG) process of graphically recording the fetal heart rate pattern and uterine contractions.

cardiovascular pertaining to the heart and blood vessels.

cardiovascular shunt an abnormal communication between chambers of the heart and/or blood vessels. In fetal life a shunt between the atria is

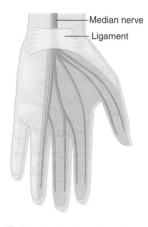

Median nerve
Ligament

■ **Figure 24** Carpal tunnel syndrome

normal to bypass the pulmonary circulation. The shunt will normally close 6–48 hours after birth.

cardiovascular system the network of passages by which blood gases and nutrients are moved around the body.

carneous pertaining to or resembling flesh.

carneous mole the appearance of a fleshy mass surrounding a dead embryo.

carotid bodies a mass of specialized epithelioid tissue containing both baroreceptors and chemoreceptors found in blood vessels in the neck. They are sensitive to fluctuating oxygen content and trigger compensatory changes in respiratory rate, heart rate and blood pressure.

carpal relating to the wrist.

carpal tunnel syndrome symptoms of altered sensation such as pain and tingling due to compression of the median nerve at the wrist (*see* Figure 24). This is usually due

to trauma but in pregnancy may be due to pressure caused by the extra fluid in the circulation.

carrier 1. a person who is physically well but harbours an infective organism and is capable of transmitting it to others. 2. an individual who carries a mutant or recessive gene without manifestation of its defective characteristic.

cartilaginous joint immovable joint composed of cartilage; this includes the sacroiliac joint and the symphysis pubis. Under the influence of oestrogen and progesterone in pregnancy these joints will soften and separate, enlarging the pelvic diameters and causing instability and movement of the pelvic girdle.

caruncle a small fleshy mass.

carunculae myrtiformes tags of tissue that remain following rupture of the hymen membranes in the vagina.

case history a record of the woman's health until her arrival at the booking clinic.

casein a protein found in milk. The casein in cows' milk is more plentiful and less digestible than that in human milk.

caseload midwifery a way of organizing midwifery practice where each midwife is responsible for the total care of a small group of women (usually between 35 and 40 per year).

cat cry syndrome (SYNONYM cri du chat syndrome) a syndrome where the newborn has a particular cry suggestive of laryngeal problems; associated with chromosome abnormalities.

cat eye syndrome vertical pupils (like those of a cat) seen in the newborn and associated with a chromosome abnormality.

catabolism metabolism by the body of complex compounds for the production of energy.

cataracts clouding or opacity of the lenses or capsule of the eyes leading to impaired vision or blindness. Congenital cataracts may be familial or associated with maternal rubella during pregnancy.

catchment area geographical region served by a specific primary health care group or hospital, including the midwife.

catecholamines a group of hormones produced in response to stress; catecholamine production in labour can inhibit progress and lead to perceived 'failure to progress'.

catgut an absorbable material made from sheep's intestine used for closure of surgical wounds.

catheter a hollow tube made from various materials which may be introduced into a cavity to achieve drainage, e.g. a *urethral catheter* for bladder drainage.

catheterization introduction of a catheter.

cathode a negative electrode.

caucasian term often used to refer to people whose skin is white or very light whose ancestors are thought to have inhabited the Caucasus region of south-eastern Europe.

cauda resembling a tail.

cauda equina the terminal branching filaments of the spinal cord which resemble a horse's tail.

caudal analgesia, caudal anaesthesia analgesia or anaesthesia achieved by injecting local anaesthetic solution into the sacral canal.

caul the amniotic membranes that have failed to rupture enclosing the infant at birth.

cautery sealing of torn blood vessels or coagulation of tissue by burning with a diathermy machine.

cavernous containing spaces or hollow areas.

cavity 1. hollow space. 2. lesion, as in dental caries.

cavity of the pelvis the region of the pelvis circumscribed by the brim, bony side walls and outlet.

CDH abbreviation for congenital dislocation of the hip.

-cele suffix denoting pathological swelling or tumour.

celiocolpotomy surgical entry into the abdomen gained through the vaginal wall.

cell a singular structural and functional unit of living organism that has the ability to grow and reproduce.

cell division a biological process of replication by mitosis, meiosis and amitosis.

cellulitis inflammation of tissue, usually the skin, due to infection or trauma.

Celsius scale scale of measurement for temperature – 0°C is freezing point and 100°C is boiling point.

census an audit or survey conducted on an entire community to measure common factors so that future service needs can be anticipated.

centi- a prefix denoting a hundredth part.

central line a fine catheter inserted into a main vein (jugular) to diagnose a condition and administer fluids or medication; used following obstetric emergency such as postpartum haemorrhage, eclampsia or DIC.

central nervous system (CNS) the brain and spinal cord.

central venous pressure (CVP) the filling pressure of the right ventricle used to regulate or monitor fluid replacement.

centre a place or group of buildings within a designated area used for providing services to the local population;

a health based unit which specializes in an aspect of care, as for example birthing centres which specialize in natural childbirth.

centre of excellence a health unit which has a particular expertise not found everywhere to which referrals and consultations can be made.

centre of gravity the midpoint or axis of rotation over which the weight of the body balances. In pregnancy the centre of gravity changes to accommodate the extra weight on the front of the abdomen; backache often results.

centrifuge an apparatus rotating at speed used for separating substances of different densities.

cephal-, cephalo- combining form meaning head.

cephalhaematoma a swelling on the neonatal head caused by a collection of blood beneath the periosteum.

cephalic presentation when the fetus adopts a head down position in the uterus the head will enter the pelvis first.

cephalic version turning of the fetus to a head presentation by internal (ICV) or external (ECV) pressure from the operator's hands.

cephalocele a congenital abnormality in which the brain tissue protrudes through incompletely formed skull bone.

cephalometry the process of measuring the head.

cephalopelvic pertaining to the relationship between the fetal head and maternal pelvis.

cephalopelvic disproportion (CPD) a mismatch between the size of the maternal pelvis and the size of the fetal head – the head is too large and will not pass through the pelvis.

cephalopelvimetry an X-ray measurement of the fetal head in relation to the pelvis to ascertain whether the head is able to pass through. Rarely used in current practice.

cerebellum the inferior part or hindbrain situated below the cerebrum and above the pons and medulla oblongata.

cerebral pertaining to or involving the cerebrum.

cerebral haemorrhage bleeding into the tissues of the brain.

cerebral palsy paralysis of various muscles and/or mental retardation as a result of damage to the brain; spasticity resulting from impaired neurological function.

cerebrospinal involving the brain and spinal cord.

cerebrospinal fluid (CSF) the fluid contained within the cerebral ventricles which bathes and cushions the brain tissues and spinal cord.

cerebrum the largest portion of the brain, occupying the upper part of the skull and consisting of left and right hemispheres.

cervical relating to the neck. In midwifery it denotes the neck of the uterus.

cervical canal the passage within the cervical muscles which permits escape of menstrual blood, entry of sperm, and passage of the baby during birth. During pregnancy it contains a thick mucus plug called the operculum.

cervical cap a contraceptive device consisting of a small rubber cap which fits tightly over the cervix to prevent the penetration of sperm.

cervical dilation the opening of the cervical canal during labour to permit the fetus to pass out of the uterus into the vaginal canal.

cervical erosion destruction of the squamous epithelial lining of the cervix by infection or trauma leaving abrasions which may bleed.

cervical polyp an overgrowth of cervical membrane forming a smooth regular mass within the cervical canal. It can also be on a stem which allows suspension into the vagina.

cervical smear scrapings of the secretions of cells from around the cervix for microscopic examination. Variations from the normal may indicate the beginning of a cancer.

cervicitis inflammation of the cervix, usually as a result of infection.

cervix lower part of the uterus which protrudes into the vagina; generally tightly closed, it will open slightly during ovulation to permit entry of sperm and at the end of the month to allow menstrual bleeding.

CESDI (Confidential Enquiry into Stillbirths and Deaths in Infancy) a government based enquiry which collects data when a baby is stillborn or dies in infancy in order to make recommendations for improving practice.

Chadwick's sign blue discoloration of the vulva and vagina as a result of venous engorgement associated with early pregnancy.

chancre the initial ulcerated lesion of syphilis formed at the site of inoculation.

Changing Childbirth Report a report published by the UK government in 1993 which contained an assessment of maternity services and recommendations for improving client satisfaction.

chi square test (GREEK *chi*, χ) a statistical test used to show the relationship between observed

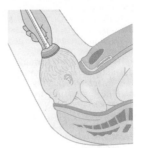

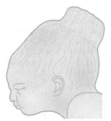

■ **Figure 25** Chignon

and expected data represented by frequencies. The test shows the probability of the data having occurred by chance.

chignon the large artificially created caput succedaneum associated with vacuum delivery (*see* Figure 25).

child a person who is of an age between birth and adolescence.

child neglect occurs where parents fail to meet the physical, social or emotional needs of the child for whom they are responsible. The child fails to thrive and social services intervene in the best interests of the child.

childbearing period the time in a woman's life between the menarche and the menopause when she is naturally capable of producing children.

childbirth preparation structured educational sessions in which a woman, her partner or a group of couples explore the meaning of childbirth and the practicalities involved.

chiropractic a therapy using manipulation to treat diseases caused by abnormal function of the nervous system and abnormality in the spinal column.

chlamydia member of the genus *Chlamydia*; a microorganism which resembles but is not a gram-negative bacterium. It can cause conjunctivitis, lymphogranuloma venereum and pelvic inflammatory disease and respiratory tract infections.

chloasma patchy hyperpigmentation often seen on the faces of pregnant women. Commonly distributed across the forehead, nose and cheeks.

choanal atresia obstruction of the posterior nasal orifices.

chocolate cyst an ovarian lesion characteristic of endometriosis in which cysts are filled with degenerated blood.

cholecystitis inflammation of the gall bladder.

chorioadenoma destruens a tumour of malignant tendency, intermediate between a hydatidiform mole and a choriocarcinoma.

chorioamnionitis inflammation of the chorionic and amnionic membranes as a result of bacterial invasion.

chorioangioma a common tumour of the placenta composed of fetal blood vessels and connective tissue in Wharton's jelly.

choriocarcinoma a fast growing tumor originating from layers of cytotrophoblast and syncytiotrophoblast. Metastases occur through the blood and lymphatic system.

chorion the outermost fetal membrane which is in contact with the uterine cavity.

chorionic gonadotrophin a water-soluble hormone originating in chorionic tissue of the blastocyst and excreted in the urine of pregnant women. Its presence is diagnostic of pregnancy.

chorionic plate the part of the fetal placenta formed by merger of the trophoblastic layer and an internal lining of mesoderm from which villi grow into the lining of the uterus in very early pregnancy.

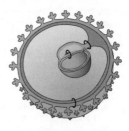

■ **Figure 26** Chorionic villi

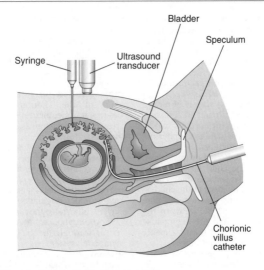

■ **Figure 27** Chorionic villus sampling

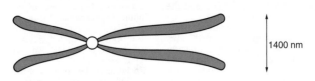

■ **Figure 28** Chromosome

chorionic villi tiny vascular projections arising from the trophoblast which grow into the maternal blood sinuses (*see* Figures 26 and 27). They absorb oxygen and nutrients to supply the demands of the growing conceptus.

choroid plexus the vascular projections which extend into the ventricles of the brain from which cerebrospinal fluid is derived.

Christmas disease a hereditary haemophilial disease resulting from deficiency of pro-coagulant Factor IX.

chromatid one of two sister chromosomes, resulting from longitudinal division in preparation for mitosis.

chromosome one of the number of microscopic structures contained in the cell nucleus which carry hereditary factors (genes) (*see* Figure 28). There are 46 in each cell, except in sperm and ovum where the number is halved.

chronic describes a condition which develops slowly and persists for a long time.

cilia hair-like cytoplasmic projections found on special

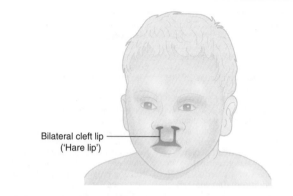

Bilateral cleft lip
('Hare lip')

■ **Figure 29** Cleft lip

epithelial cells; they beat rhythmically causing a current and enabling propulsion.

circulation movement in a defined circuit, e.g. *circulation of the blood.*

circulatory system the closed circuit or network of blood vessels, heart and lungs which supply the tissues of the body with all they need, remove waste, and carry micro-organisms, cancer cells and drugs.

circumcision term applying to mutilation of the genitals in either gender, often in the first few days of life. In males, the excision of the foreskin or pre-puce of the penis. Carried out as a religious and cultural practice on the 8th day of life by Jews and Muslims; carries physical and psychological risks.

circumvallate surrounded by an elevation, as in *circumvallate placenta,* a placenta in which an overgrowth of chorionic membranes results in formation of a white ridge about the circumference.

clamp an instrument used to compress vessels or hollow organs to prevent bleeding, e.g. a *cord clamp* is used to clamp the umbilical cord after birth.

classic caesarean section delivery of the baby through a vertical incision made into the abdomen and the upper segment of the uterus. Repair and recovery are more difficult; in future labours the mother may be at greater risk of uterine rupture.

clavicle the collar bone, a long bone between the sternum and the scapula. It may break or be broken (cleidotomy) if shoulder dystocia occurs in the second stage of labour.

cleft division or fissure.

cleft lip (hare lip) congenital defect resulting from failure of embryonic fusion of the median nasal and maxillary processes (*see* Figure 29 and Figure 62).

cleft palate congenital defect which usually accompanies cleft lip. The fissure may be partial or complete allowing communication between oral and nasal passage. The hard palate and gums may be absent or twisted.

cleidotomy breaking of the clavicle at the sternoclavicular joint to facilitate delivery of the fetus where there is obstruction due to the shoulders being too large.

climacteric the change of life; the menopause.

clinic a place with limited medical equipment where patients not requiring hospitalization can be seen by, obtain advice from, or be screened by a professionally qualified person.

clinical assessment the evaluation of a person's physical condition; the theoretical application of knowledge to practice.

clitoridectomy the removal of part or all of the clitoris. In many countries it is ritually performed on pubescent girls. In the UK it is considered to be an act of genital mutilation, is forbidden by law and as such is a basis for granting asylum status.

clitoris female erectile tissue, situated externally at the anterior junction of the labia minora and internally around the walls of the vagina. Once thought to be a homologue of the male penis, now known to be much larger and more intricate than previously realized.

clone a group of cells which are genetically identical, individually created by asexual reproduction and having identical genetic make-up.

clonic a term applied to the rapid involuntary muscular contraction and relaxation seen in seizures or fits.

clostridium a bacterium of the genus *Clostridium*, a group of spore-forming anaerobic bacteria which cause gangrene, botulism, cellulitis and tetanus.

clot solidification of blood.

clotting time the time required for shed blood to clot under normal conditions.

club foot (talipes) a congenital malformation in which the foot is inverted and rotated.

CNS abbreviation for central nervous system.

coagulate to change from a liquid to jelly-like mass.

coagulation clumping together of red blood cells.

coagulation factor one of the 12 substances in the blood which are required for the formation of a blood clot.

cocaine baby a baby born to a mother who has used cocaine during pregnancy and which is showing signs of withdrawal.

coccus (PLURAL cocci) grain or seed – used to describe a microorganism of similar characteristic shape.

coccygeal relating to the coccyx.

coccygeus one of the muscles of the pelvic floor arising from the ischial spines and anchored into the lateral borders of the sacrum and coccyx.

coccyx the lowest bone of the spinal column, formed by the fusion of four rudimentary vertebrae.

Cochrane Database information from an institution which collates and reviews quantitative research on maternity care.

cohort a group of people with characteristics in common used for research enquiry.

cohort study examination of the characteristics of a group of people, usually over time, to develop new knowledge.

coitus sexual intercourse; copulation.

colic acute spasmodic abdominal pain. In infancy it can be due to overfeeding or swallowing of air resulting in bouts of crying.

cold injury cellular damage and impaired function occurring as a result of exposure to cold environmental temperatures.

collapse a state of deep depression or exhaustion causing a person to be unable to function.

collodion baby a baby born with skin resembling a scaly paper-like membrane.

colostrum the first milk secreted by the breasts. It contains large quantities of cells, lactalbumin and lactoprotein.

colovaginal pertaining to the colon and vagina, as in *colovaginal fistula*, a fistula or abnormal opening between the two structures.

colpalgia pain in the vagina.

colpocystitis inflammation of the vagina and urinary bladder.

colpocystocele protrusion of the urinary bladder into the vagina, usually through a weakness or fistula in the anterior vaginal wall.

colporrhaphy surgical suturing and repair of the vaginal wall.

colposcope an instrument with a lens and a light used to examine the vagina and cervix; a vaginal speculum.

colpotomy a surgical incision into the wall of the vagina.

communicating hydrocephalus hydrocephalus in which there is ventricular communication due to either excess or extra cerebrospinal fluid being produced or poorly reabsorbed.

compatibility the ability to coexist harmoniously.

compensation the process of increasing efficiency in one physiologic structure to restore balance to a system, structure or body when another aspect of that system has failed.

competence the ability to perform actions or procedures to an acceptable standard, befitting that for which one has been trained.

competences (competencies) statements accepted by professional midwifery organizations throughout Europe (although definitions are also set at a wider level) which describe in detail skills a trained midwife is able to perform and towards which a student midwife is working.

complementary feeds feeds given to a neonate in addition to planned feeding regimen, whether breast or bottle feeds.

complementary therapy therapies and treatments which do not follow a Western health care model but which can be used in conjunction with this approach. Examples include reflexology, herbal medicines, psychoprophylaxis, osteopathy, cranial osteopathy, relaxation therapy and acupuncture.

complete abortion the total expulsion of all products of conception.

complete breech the fetus is lying with the knees and hips flexed or folded up and the buttocks presenting over the cervical os.

complicated labour a labour in which there is a departure from the normal progress.

complication a deviation from the normal or expected process.

compound presentation a complication of labour in which more than one part of the fetus presents and may create an obstruction, e.g. head or arm.

concealed haemorrhage bleeding which is not obvious or which cannot be seen, but which will cause deterioration in the condition of the individual and the vital signs.

conception 1. the mental, abstract formulation of ideas. 2. the fertilization of the ovum by a spermatozoon.

conceptional age the age of the fetus or embryo in weeks from conception rather than from the last menstrual period – usually 2 weeks less.

■ Figure 30 Condom

conceptus refers to the fertilized ovum from the uniting of the gametes until delivery.

condensed milk cows' milk which has been concentrated by removal of at least one third of the water and to which sugar has been added. Not suitable to feed to newborn babies.

condom a protective rubber sheath worn over the penis during sexual intercourse for preventing conception and cross-infection, especially with HIV (*see* Figure 30).

confidential enquiry all cases of maternal death in the UK are reviewed and conclusions from the reviews published at 3-yearly intervals. Avoidable factors contributing to the death are identified and recommendations for practice made.

confinement 1. detention. 2. the period of childbearing or labour and the puerperium.

confluence of the sinuses the wide junction or point of merger of the superior sagittal, straight and occipital sinuses with the large transverse sinuses. Trauma to the head from forceps, assisted breech delivery or abnormal moulding may cause bleeding into the brain and cerebral palsy may result.

congenital present at birth.

congenital dislocation of the hip (CDH) condition existing at birth where the hip joint is lax or the socket in which the head of femur sits is shallow and the hips dislocate easily. Diagnosed by Barlow's test for hip instability and treated with splints.

congenital syphilis infection of a baby in utero due to placental transfer of the causative organism from a woman who has had syphilis during pregnancy. The neonate will have specific characteristics and be mentally retarded.

congestive dysmenorrhoea painful periods caused by extra blood in the vessels of the pelvis.

conjoined manipulation the use of both hands, coming together from different points for certain procedures.

conjoined twins multiple pregnancy in which there has been incomplete cleavage of a single fertilized ovum. The twins remain partially joined together.

conjugata to bind or act together; referring to the conjugate diameters of the pelvis.

conjunctivitis inflammation of the mucous membrane lining the anterior aspect of the eyes and eyelids. In the neonate it may be due to infection acquired during passage through the vagina.

consanguinity a blood relationship between two people who then conceive a child.

consent clients must give permission for tests and treatment to be carried out on them. Midwives have a statutory obligation to inform clients of

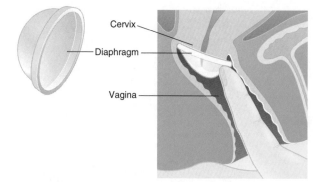

Figure 31 Contraceptive diaphragm

available tests and treatment including the side-effects of each. The client must be of sound mind, able to absorb the information and make a decision as to what care she requires. If she desires to have a particular procedure, she will then give verbal or written informed consent.

constipation inability to evacuate stools despite feeling the desire to do so.

constriction ring a spasmodic contraction of uterine muscles leading to narrowing, usually at the junction of the upper and lower segments.

contamination exposure of a sterile or clean fluid, tissue or person to pathogenic organisms.

continuous positive airway pressure (CPAP) non-invasive ventilation in which the flow of air is delivered at a constant pressure preventing complete collapse of the alveoli after each expiration as happens in babies with respiratory distress syndrome.

contraception the prevention of conception.

contraceptive diaphragm a large rubber dome with a compressible outer ring which can be inserted into the vagina with spermicidal cream to prevent conception (*see* Figure 31).

contraceptive method a measure designed to prevent sperm meeting ovum. Many methods are available and different methods suit different people.

contracted pelvis a pelvis in which any of the diameters are sufficiently shortened to interfere with the progress of labour.

contraction temporary shortening of muscle fibres. In labour this is accompanied by a degree of permanent muscle shortening during subsequent relaxation, retraction.

contraction stress test (CST) an artificial stimulation of contraction of the uterus using oxytocin and simultaneous electronic monitoring of the fetal heart, unrelated to labour. The fetal response is assessed as an indicator of its ability to withstand the rigours of labour.

control of haemorrhage measures to arrest bleeding from the genital tract so that deterioration in the condition of the mother does not occur. Can be achieved by active

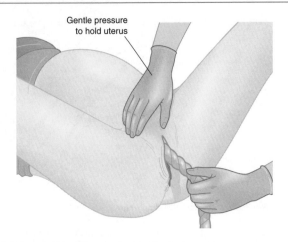

Gentle pressure
to hold uterus

■ **Figure 32** Controlled cord traction

management of the third stage of labour.

controlled cord traction method of delivering the placenta and membranes by putting tension on the umbilical cord after an oxytocic drug has been given by injection and the uterus contracted (*see* Figure 32).

controlled drug a pharmaceutical preparation whose prescription, administration, storage, dose, frequency of use and disposal is prescribed by statute because the drug may be misused or cause addiction.

convulsion an involuntary, generalized spasm of voluntary muscle fibres.

Cooley's anaemia thalassaemia.

Coombs' test test performed on cord blood to detect the presence of antibodies on the red cell surface. It is an indication of fetal/maternal incompatibility.

cord blood blood is taken from the umbilical vein or/and artery just after delivery to perform blood gases and do diagnostic tests.

cord presentation the umbilical cord is presenting at the cervical os; continuation of labour may cause the fetal circulation to be impeded, with potentially fatal results (*see* Figure 33).

cord prolapse the umbilical cord prolapses through the cervical os into the vagina (and possibly out of the introitus). A potentially fatal condition for the baby which is usually treated by holding the presenting part up, thereby taking pressure off the cord, and offering immediate caesarean section (*see* Figure 34).

cornu (SYNONYM horn) the junction of the fallopian tubes with the uterus.

cornual pregnancy a pregnancy which has implanted in the narrow section of the fallopian tube as it enters the uterus. The pregnancy is not viable as the tube will rupture with severe bleeding by week 12 – this is an emergency

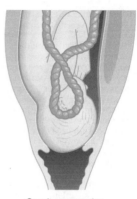

Presentation
of the cord

Occult presentation
of the cord

■ **Figure 33** Cord presentation

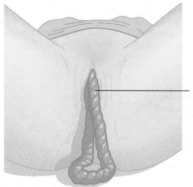

Prolapsed cord
at the vulva

■ **Figure 34** Cord prolapse

life-threatening situation requiring urgent surgery.

coronal suture the soft, fibrous, membranous region on the fetal skull between the frontal and parietal bones on each side of the skull.

corpus (SYNONYM body) the *corpus albicans* is the place on the ovary which has healed since the ovum escaped and the *corpus luteum* (formed after ovulation to produce oestrogen and progesterone) degenerated and stopped producing hormones.

corpus cavernosum spongy tissue in the penis or clitoris which becomes distended with blood during sexual arousal.

corpus luteum the yellow, blister-like follicle found on the surface of the ovary after expulsion of the ovum. It lives a short time and produces endocrine hormones; however, if pregnancy occurs its life is extended by the influence of human chorionic gonadotrophin.

cortex outermost layer of an organ.

cortisone one of several hormones produced by the adrenal cortex.

cot death the unexplained death of an infant (*see under* sudden infant death syndrome).

cotyledon a lobe or distantly separated group of placental villi supplied with blood vessels and supported by membranes.

course a programme of learning experiences designed to enable participants to meet objectives set by a validating authority (e.g. a college or university).

couvade the mock labour sometimes experienced by men when their partner is in labour.

Couvelaire uterus bruised and purplish-blue discoloration of the uterus caused by blood escaping between the myometrial fibres. It is unable to contract because of the volume of blood within the tissues and so the placental site will continue to bleed unchecked.

crack baby an infant exposed to the effects of cocaine in pregnancy.

cracked nipples associated with breastfeeding. The baby is not positioned correctly and the gums chew the lower margins of the nipple causing pain, cracking and bleeding. The baby will not get milk and will become hungry and frustrated.

cradle cap thick, yellow, greasy scales on the scalp of the infant.

cranial bones the bones of the skull (*see* Figure 35).

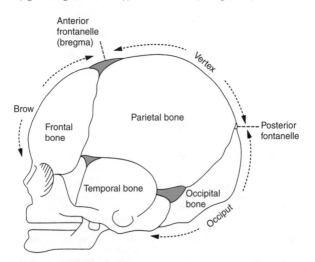

■ **Figure 35 Cranial bones**

cranial suture the fibromem-branous structure found between the bones of the cranium in infancy.

craniodidymus a form of conjoined twins with two heads but fused bodies.

craniotabes defects and depressions found in the bones of the skull as the depositing of calcium in fetal life has not kept pace with cerebral development.

cranium skull.

Credé's expression a rarely used method of assisting placental expulsion in which the uterine fundus is massaged to stimulate contraction, then squeezed.

cretinism a congenital condition in which the thyroid is deficient and a set of recognizable features are present including dwarfism and mental retardation.

cri du chat kitten-type mewing cry heard in the infant with neurological damage.

cricoid pressure pressure applied to the cartilage of the larynx during induction of anaesthesia to protect the airway from gastric reflux.

criterion a standard which must be met and against which other standards or practices can be judged.

cross-infection the passing of pathogenic organisms from an infected person to a healthy one.

cross-matching of blood the procedure by which a donor's blood is mixed with that of a potential recipient to ensure compatibility before a blood transfusion.

crowning when the suboccipi-tobregmatic and biparietal diameters of the fetal head distend the vulva and the head no longer recedes between contractions during the second stage of labour (*see* Figure 36).

crown–rump length (CRL) ultrasonic measurement taken of the fetus during the first

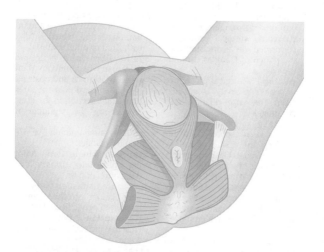

■ **Figure 36** Crowning

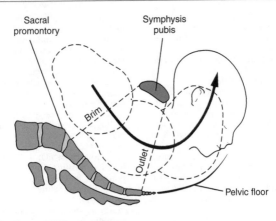

Figure 37 Curve of Carus

trimester to assess gestational age.

cryptodidymus conjoined twins, one being considerable smaller and developing within the body of the other.

culdocentesis removal of intraperitoneal fluids by aspiration with a hollow needle introduced through the vagina.

culdotomy surgical procedure performed via an incision into the pouch of Douglas through the vagina.

curettage a surgical procedure in which a cavity is scraped clean (*see also* dilation and curettage).

curette a surgical instrument like a small spoon used for scraping the inside of hollow organs; used to clean the uterus of products of conception.

curriculum vitae (CV) a summary of a person's education, qualifications, professional experience, honours and activities sent to a prospective employer. (*See* Appendix.)

curve of Carus name given to the direction or pathway in which the fetal head moves to

pass through the pelvis (*see* Figure 37).

cutaneous relating to the skin.

cyanosis blue discoloration of the skin and mucous membranes due to deficient oxygenation.

cyesis pregnancy.

cyst an enclosed pouch within tissue or organ, having a membranous lining, which is filled with fluid or other material.

cystic fibrosis a congenital disease in which mucous gland secretion is thick and obstructive. Malabsorption in the intestines and infection in the lungs are among the predominant features.

cystitis inflammation of the urinary bladder.

cysto- combining form denoting gall bladder, urinary bladder, pouch or cyst.

cystocele herniation of the urinary bladder into the vagina as a result of pelvic floor damage.

cytogenetics a branch of science in which cells and chromosomes are studied.

cytomegalovirus (CMV) a virus closely related to herpes.

Infection of the fetus in utero may cause cytomegalic inclusion disease and result in an infant that may be small for gestational age, jaundiced and suffer from liver disease.

cytoplasm the protoplasm of a cell other than the nucleus.

cytotoxic drug strong drug or chemical agent used to kill cancerous cells in the body. Such drug exposure during pregnancy will cause congenital abnormalities.

cytotrophoblast the inner cellular layer of the trophoblast.

Dd

D, d symbol denoting rhesus blood group, others being C, c and E, e.

D&C (dilation and curettage) dilation of the cervix and scraping out (curettage) of the uterine lining. Used to evacuate products of conception following incomplete abortion or as a diagnostic and therapeutic procedure in gynaecology (*see* Figure 41, below).

dactyl digit.

Dangerous Drugs Act (DDA) Act of Parliament regulating the manufacture, distribution and use of habit-forming drugs. Replaced by the Misuse of Drugs Act 1971.

day assessment unit a place where screening and diagnosis can be done without the woman needing to stay overnight.

dead fetus syndrome a dead fetus is retained in utero; if delivery does not occur the decomposition of the fetus may lead to blood coagulation disorders and severe haemorrhage at delivery.

deceleration slowing down. In *fetal heart deceleration* the fetal heart rate falls to below 90 beats per minute (b.p.m.) from a normal baseline rate of 120–150 b.p.m. (*see* Figure 38).

decidua the lining of the uterus during pregnancy.

decidua basalis the part of the decidua beneath the implanted ovum.

decidua capsularis the part of the decidua which covers the implanted ovum.

decidual endometritis inflammation or infection of the decidua during pregnancy.

deciduoma a benign or malignant tumour in the endometrial tissue.

decrement a decrease in or decline in frequency or efficiency.

deep transverse arrest the fetal head is unable to pass through the pelvis. It enters but cannot rotate or descend further.

deep vein thrombosis a blood clot forms in the muscle of the leg, usually the calf. Pregnant women are at risk due to changes in clotting mechanism and immobility in labour or at caesarean section.

defaecation the act of emptying the bowel.

deflexion a turning to one side; attitude of the fetal head when partially flexed.

deflower the tearing of the hymen membrane over the vaginal orifice, usually at first intercourse; loss of virginity.

deformity the condition of being distorted, flawed, malformed or misshapen.

degeneration destruction of cells resulting in impaired function.

degree 1. a unit of mathematical measurement, e.g. of temperature. 2. one of the intervals on a measuring tool, e.g. a thermometer. 3. an academic award conferred by a university or college.

dehiscence splitting open, as in the breaking down of a wound.

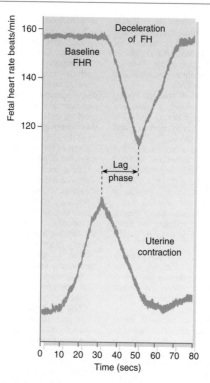

■ **Figure 38** Deceleration of fetal heart seen on cardiograph

dehydration excessive loss of water from the body.

delay in labour prolongation of any of the three stages of labour.

delayed postpartum haemorrhage (SYNONYM secondary postpartum haemorrhage) severe bleeding from the genital tract 24 hours after childbirth, usually due to retained products of conception preventing uterine contraction.

delivery the expulsion of the fetus, placenta and membranes.

delusion a false belief held by a person despite evidence against it.

demand feeding feeding the baby as and when it seems to be hungry, rather than at set times.

Demerol® trade name for meperidine, a narcotic analgesic similar to pethidine.

demography the study of populations and the incidence of disease, infection, etc.

denominator a defined point of the presenting part of the fetus which in relation to a given point on the mother's pelvis is used to indicate its position, occiput, mentum or sacrum.

deoxyribonucleic acid (DNA) a complex nucleoprotein found in chromosomes bearing coded genetic information and capable of reproduction in the presence of the appropriate enzyme (*see* Figure 42, below).

Department of Health (DoH) the government department which administers the UK National Health Service and sanctions policies.

dependence a state of being unable to function without that on which dependence is founded, e.g. a drug; a state of being reliant upon a person or substance.

depressant a drug which depresses or reduces the functioning of a system or of the whole body.

depression 1. a hollow or fossa. 2. a lowering of mood or state resulting in extreme sadness or dejection in which the person may be unable to carry out daily functions.

deprivation a state of being without the necessities for optimal physical, mental, social or spiritual well-being.

dermal referring to the skin or cutaneous layer.

dermoid cyst a benign cystic swelling containing skin and hair.

descent a movement downward. The term is applied to the presenting part of the fetus as it moves through the pelvis towards the outlet. Assessed frequently in labour as it is an indicator of progress.

detachment separation or loss of anchorage of a structure from its support.

detrusor urinae muscle important fibres that form the outer layer of the urinary bladder. Because of the proximity to the vagina damage can occur during childbirth which can result in incontinence.

development process of change and adaptation to a more advanced level of functioning. *Developmental age* is an expression of a child's age when compared to a standard measurement.

developmental anomaly any abnormality or defect occurring before birth.

developmental horizon any of the 25 stages of development of the human embryo.

deviant a person who does not follow socially accepted standards or behaviour.

deviant behaviour actions contrary to those done by the majority of the community or culture.

deviation variation or turning away from a regular course or expected position.

deviation from normal a clinical finding commonly regarded as contrary to the normal or expected findings. The Midwives Code of Conduct requests that the midwife report such findings to a medical practitioner.

dexamethasone a corticosteroid given to women in premature labour which facilitates lung maturation and reduces the risk of RDS in the neonate.

dextral referring to the right side.

dextran a high molecular weight, water-soluble polysaccharide purified preparation which is used as a plasma expander for maintaining blood pressure and emergency treatment of shock.

dextro-, dextr- a combining term meaning favouring or turning to the right.

dextrocardia the heart is in the right half of the chest rather than the left.

dextrose a monosaccharide or sugar, the simplest form of carbohydrate.

di- prefix meaning two, twice.

diabetes insipidus a disease characterized by deficiency of antidiuretic hormone (vasopressin) resulting in excessive thirst and excretion of excessive volumes of dilute urine.

diabetes mellitus a disease with familial tendency in which there is defective metabolism of carbohydrates due to reduction in the secretion of insulin. Characteristic presentation is hyperglycaemia, glycosuria, polyuria, polydipsia, weight loss and ketoacidosis. Women with diabetes are at risk of infertility, abortion, intrauterine death, macrosomic infants, pregnancy-induced hypertension (PIH) and shoulder dystocia.

diabetic acidosis metabolic acidosis of uncontrolled diabetes in which there is an excess production of ketone bodies resulting from metabolism of body fats.

diagnosis identification of disease based on assessment of clinical symptoms.

diagnostic process systems used to indicate the nature of disease; follows on from a screening test.

diagonal any plane or straight line that is not vertical, perpendicular or horizontal; slantwise.

diagonal conjugate measurement of the internal pelvis, taken from the sacral promontory to the lower border of the symphysis pubis. In the normal pelvis it should measure 12.5 cm.

diameter a straight line passing through the centre of an object that joins points which go from one side to the other side of an organ, the pelvis or the fetal head.

diameters of fetal skull distances between certain landmarks on the fetal skull (*see* Figure 39). Used to determine whether or not the head is able to pass through the pelvis.

diaphragm 1. a muscular partition which separates the chest and abdomen and is a major muscle of respiration. 2. a contraceptive device made of domed rubber over a compressible outer ring. When inserted into the vault of the vagina it covers the cervix preventing the passage of sperm.

diaphragmatic hernia embryonic development of the diaphragm in which there is persistence of the pleuroperitoneal

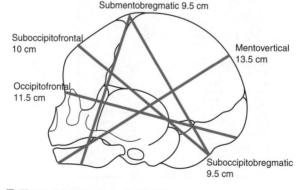

Submentobregmatic 9.5 cm

Suboccipitofrontal 10 cm

Mentovertical 13.5 cm

Occipitofrontal 11.5 cm

Suboccipitobregmatic 9.5 cm

■ Figure 39 Diameters of fetal skull

canal allowing part of the bowel to pass into the chest cavity (*see* Figure 40).

diarrhoea frequent passage of loose, watery stools; often caused by a gastrointestinal infection.

diastasis separation of parts normally joined together, e.g. *symphysis pubis diastasis*.

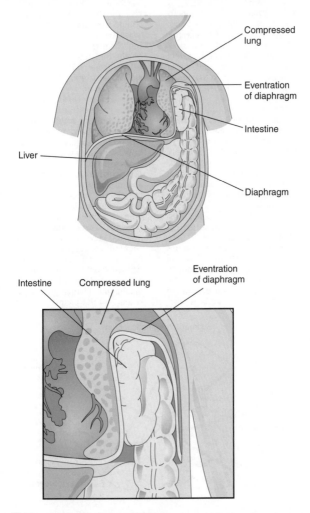

■ **Figure 40** Diaphragmatic hernia

diastole the resting phase of the cardiac cycle during which the chambers of the heart are dilated and fill with blood.

diastolic blood pressure the minimal measured pressure of blood felt in peripheral vessels during ventricular resting phase.

diathermy the applied therapeutic use of heat produced by high frequency current to body tissue. Used to seal tissue together including bleeding vessels.

diazepam (Valium) a tranquillizer used in management of fits.

DIC *see* disseminated intravascular coagulation.

dicephalus a fetus with two heads.

didactylism only two digits on each hand.

didymus a testis.

diet the food which one eats.

dietician a health professional concerned with advising people about their eating patterns and offering nutritional advice.

differential diagnosis examination and comparison of signs and symptoms to distinguish between diseases of similar characteristics.

differentiation unspecified cells are modified and organized to have specific characteristics and perform specific functions.

diffusion substances pass through a semi-permeable membrane from an area of high concentration to one of low concentration.

digestion the process of breaking down into smaller parts or simpler compounds; the action of enzymes on ingested foods.

digestive juices enzymes found in the mouth and stomach which break down food. In pregnancy the stomach enzymes are more acidic than at other times and, if regurgitated, can cause burning of the mucous linings of the oesophagus (*see* Mendelson's syndrome).

digit a finger or toe.

dilatation (SYNONYM dilation) the process of stretching and opening, usually of a sphincter but also the cervix during labour.

dilation and curettage (D&C) widening of the cervix and scraping out of the contents of the uterus; used as a diagnostic and therapeutic procedure in obstetrics and gynaecology (*see* Figure 41).

diplococci (SINGULAR diplococcus) descriptive appearance of micrococci that always form pairs.

dimorphism having the appearance of both sexes.

diovulatory two ova are released during one menstrual cycle.

diphtheria a rare but acute and potentially fatal infection against which a vaccine is offered during the first weeks of life.

diphtheria toxoid, tetanus toxoid and pertussis vaccine (DTP) combined immunization offered in the first few weeks of life.

diploid having double quantities. Chromosomes have diploid numbers or 23 pairs.

diplopagus conjoined twins which are equally developed.

direct Coombs' test *see* Coombs' test.

direct endometriosis invasion of the myometrium by the mucous membranes lining the uterus.

disability a restriction in a person's ability to behave in a manner or within the range considered by the majority of the population as normal.

disaccharide a carbohydrate formed by condensation of two simple sugars.

disadvantaged a group of people who lack money or resources considered standard

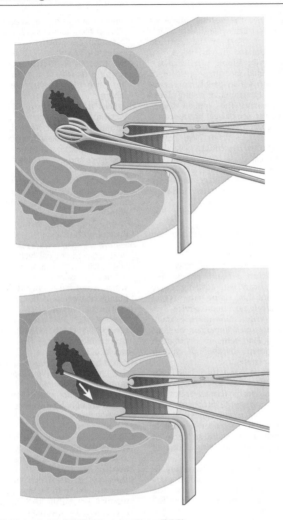

■ Figure 41 Dilation and curettage (D&C)

or normal by the majority of people.

discharge to emit, dismiss or release.

discharge summary report of events during hospitalization sent to a person's general practitioner.

disease an abnormal condition caused by injury, infection or cancer resulting in a disturbance of normal bodily function.

disengagement emergence from a contained space; the manual removal of the fetal head or presenting part from the pelvis during caesarean section.

disinfect to destroy microorganisms by applying strong fluids or chemicals.

disjunction 1. moving apart or separation. 2. separation of homologous chromosomes at meiosis or mitotic division.

dislocation displacement of bone from its original position.

disproportion lack of fit between two objects, for example referring to the relationship in which the fetal head is too large to pass through the maternal pelvis.

disseminated intravascular coagulation (DIC) a condition in which there is widespread consumption of clotting factors and failure of haemostasis. It is a complication associated with pregnancy-induced hypertension (PIH) or severe haemorrhage.

distress suffering; exhaustion; in danger; a level of stress/stimulation considered to be detrimental to health.

diuresis increased secretion of urine.

dizygotic twins two fetuses in the same pregnancy developed from two ova released simultaneously.

DNA abbreviation of deoxyribonucleic acid. The substance found in the chromosomes of nucleus which carries coded genetic information and is capable of reproduction (*see* Figure 42).

DNA testing examination of the deoxyribonucleic acid (DNA). Can detect inherited

disease carriers and determine paternity.

Döderlein's bacillus (*Lactobacillus acidophilus*) a gram-positive bacillus which is a normal inhabitant of the vagina. These bacilli digest glucose to form lactic acid which protects against infection.

dominance expression of control.

dominant gene term applied to the one gene out of two genes which will shape the future individual. The capacity of one gene to exert control or express its characteristic trait in the presence of a similar gene.

dominant inheritance a hereditary pattern in which one gene of a pair overrules the characteristic expression of the other.

'domino' scheme a woman has her baby in hospital cared for by the community midwife. She will return home 6 hours after giving birth.

donor one who gives blood or tissue to another.

Doppler ultrasound scanning a procedure used to assess the flow of blood through vessels; Doppler scanning is used to visualize the flow of fetal blood through the umbilical vessels.

dorsal referring to the posterior part of an organ.

dose the measured quantity of a medicine to be given at any one time.

double-blind trial a research study in which an intervention is administered to one proportion of the sample and a placebo to the other but neither the subjects nor the administrators know which group are receiving active intervention thereby avoiding subjectivity and removing potential bias.

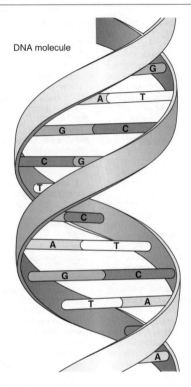

DNA molecule

■ **Figure 42** DNA molecule

douche washing, lavage, using a stream of water, usually applied to the genitals.

doula a lay person or birth attendant who provides non-clinical support and advocacy to another woman throughout labour. Doulas may also provide postnatal support.

Down's syndrome (SYNONYM trisomy 21) a congenital defect of chromosome resulting in variable level of mental retardation. An extra chromosome 21 is present. Older mothers are considered most at risk and screening tests are available to estimate the risk.

drug a chemical compound given to change the responses of the body to its environment, substance used for medical purposes.

drug abuse substances are introduced into the body other than for therapeutic use; over-use of a drug for enhanced stimulant, hallucinogenic or other non-therapeutic effect that results in addiction.

drug addiction the inability of the individual to function without certain substances in their blood.

drug concentration the measurable amount of a substance in the blood when tested to determine uptake and to guide further therapeutic administration.

drug-induced teratogenesis a congenital abnormality resulting from the absorption of a certain substance which alters genetic coding and cellular development in the fetus.

drug resistance the lack of sensitivity or expected response to a therapeutic preparation; the ability of micro-organisms to withstand the effect of an antibiotic substance.

drug tolerance the gradually acquired ability to resist the effect of a drug; acquired insensitivity; the requirement to increase the dose of a drug regularly to maintain the same effect.

dry labour colloquial term used to describe labour when there is no leakage of liquor amnii, the membranes having ruptured before the onset of labour.

Dubowitz score an assessment devised for determining gestational age of infants based on several physical and behavioural characteristics. (*See* Appendix.)

duct a tube conveying secretions away from source.

ductus arteriosus a bypass blood vessel that shunts blood between the left pulmonary artery and the aorta in fetal life; it normally closes at birth.

ductus venosus a venous channel in the fetus, the umbilical vein passing through the liver and joining into the inferior vena cava.

duplex having two parts.

dura mater toughened fibromembranous lining of the skull, forming the outermost covering of the brain tissue and spinal cord.

dural tap a complication of the epidural procedure in which cerebrospinal fluid leaks. Severe headache occurs and lasts several days.

Dutch cap *see* diaphragm.

duty of care the requirement on a professionally trained person to behave in a prescribed manner.

dwarfism abnormally short stature caused by either genetic alteration, endocrine conditions or chronic disease.

dys- prefix, meaning disordered, abnormal, difficult or painful.

dysfunctional uterine bleeding bleeding from the uterus not associated with pregnancy, tumour or menstruation.

dyskaryosis irregularity in nuclear shape or number.

dysmaturity the failure of an organism or fetus to achieve expected development. This term may be applied to a fetus that is small for gestational age or one that is large for gestational age but whose behaviour is immature.

dysmenorrhoea difficult or painful menstruation.

dysmorphia deformity.

dyspareunia difficult or painful coitus.

dyspnoea difficult or laboured breathing.

dystocia difficult or problematic labour. In *shoulder dystocia*, the head delivers but the shoulders fail to be delivered easily during the second stage of labour.

dysuria difficult or painful urination.

Ee

E, e symbol used to denote rhesus blood types, others being C, c and D, d.

E. coli (*Escherichia coli*) a gramnegative bacterium which normally inhabits the intestine. Outside of the intestinal tract it causes infection.

Ebstein's anomaly a congenital heart condition in which the tricuspid valve is located deep into the right ventricle creating obstruction to filling and other symptoms including heart failure.

ecboline an abortifacient or substance used for accelerating labour.

ecchymosis bruising caused by leakage of blood into the subcutaneous tissue.

ECG (electrocardiogram) a measurement of the electrical activity in the heart during contraction which can be recorded in graphic form.

echoencephalography pulsed echo or ultrasound used to examine the intracranial structures.

eclampsia seizure or convulsion associated with pregnancy in which the blood pressure rises rapidly and there is oedema and proteinuria.

ecto- combining form meaning outside or out of place, as in *ectopic pregnancy*.

ectoderm the outermost of the three primary germinal layers of the embryo.

-ectomy combining form meaning surgical cutting away of tissue.

ectopic not in the normal position.

ectopic pregnancy pregnancy developing outside of the uterine cavity, usually in the fallopian tube but sometimes in the abdominal cavity (*see* Figure 43). The pregnancy outgrows the blood supply by 10 weeks and erodes blood vessels which bleed creating an obstetric emergency.

ectrodactyly a congenital condition in which there is absence of one or more fingers or toes or parts of them.

ectropion eversion of a part, e.g. the eyelid or cervix.

eczema an inflammatory condition of the skin characterized by combination of itching, redness, scaling and production of exudate. Usually congenital but may be set off by artificial feeding in sensitive babies.

education a change in behaviour resulting from reflecting on a range of designed experiences.

EEG *see* electroencephalogram.

effacement loss of form of the uterine cervix during labour (*see* Figure 44).

efferent carrying or conducting away from centre to peripheries.

effusion the pouring out of any fluid into surrounding tissue or cavity.

ejaculation 1. sudden explosion or emission. 2. release of semen.

elasticity the characteristic of being able to stretch and return to original shape. *Elastic*

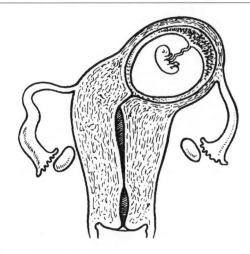

Figure 43 Ectopic pregnancy

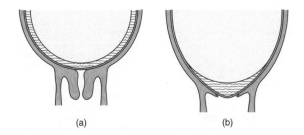

(a)   (b)

Figure 44 Effacement of cervix

stockings are knee-high or thigh-high self-retaining stockings applied before surgery, e.g. caesarean section, to prevent pooling of blood in the legs thereby reducing the risk of thrombosis occurring.

elderly primigravida colloquial term describing a woman over the age of 35 years in her first pregnancy; carries little real meaning in clinical terms except that ascribed to it by some practitioners.

elective done by choice; *elective surgery* is planned surgery which is neither urgent nor mandatory.

elective caesarean section caesarean section done at a time and date of choice with no immediate danger to the life of the fetus or mother; may be done to avoid a potential complication of labour.

electrocardiogram (ECG) a graphical record of electrical impulses emitted by the heart during a cardiac cycle.

electrode a conductor transmitting an electrical wave from its source to another medium or instrument. Fetal scalp electrodes are attached to the fetal scalp and record the heart activity on a printout.

electroencephalogram (EEG) a graphic record of electrical waves emitted by the cerebral cortex.

electrolyte a substance which in solution is capable of conducting electrical current.

electrolyte balance the balance between the salts, sodium, potassium, chlorides in the bodily fluids.

electrolyte solution a fluid which is capable of conducting an electric current.

electronic fetal monitor (EFM) a method of recording fetal heart activity by applying an electrode to the scalp. Uterine activity is recorded at the same time. The machine to which the electrode is attached can make the pulse audible and transmit it as a graphic record on paper.

elimination the process of expelling the waste products of the body.

embolism the occlusion of a blood vessel by particulate, clots, air, amniotic fluid or foreign body which travels from another part of the body, e.g. *pulmonary embolism*.

embolus a foreign body, air, gas, tumour, liquor or clot of blood which moves around the circulation.

embryectomy surgical removal of an extrauterine embryo, as is done following an ectopic pregnancy.

embryo the early stage of development – from fertilization to the end of the 8th week of gestation (*see* Figure 45).

embryo transfer a procedure whereby an ovum fertilized in the laboratory is introduced into the uterus.

embryology the scientific study of early human development.

embryonal carcinoma a cancer of embryonic cells.

embryonic abortion termination of a pregnancy before the 12th week of gestation.

embryonic disc the three-layer plate of cells from which the embryo develops in the 2nd week of pregnancy (*see* Figure 46).

embryonic stage the stage of pregnancy from the end of the germinal stage 10th day, until the end of the 8th week.

embryotomy intentional destruction of an embryo in utero to facilitate removal when natural delivery is impossible.

emergency sudden development of pathological condition which requires immediate medical attention if survival is to be ensured.

emesis the act of vomiting.

eminence a projection, prominent part of a bone.

Emmet's operation surgical repair of a perineal or cervical tear.

emollient a substance which softens tissue or soothes an inflammation.

emotion psychologic strong feelings often accompanied by outward expression of mood change.

emotional deprivation absence of affection, regard, interest or encouragement of one person towards another, usually a parent for a child.

empathy ability to understand the feelings or emotions of another person.

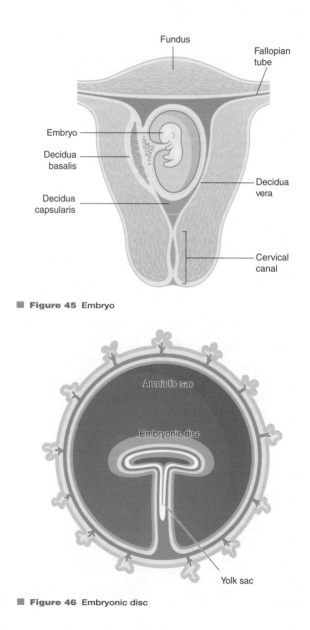

Figure 45 Embryo

Figure 46 Embryonic disc

empowerment the process by which midwives (and others) should enable women to feel that they can make their own decisions and choices, based on all available knowledge and without being influenced by others.

empty follicle syndrome a condition in which there are no oocytes in a graafian follicle.

encephalin (enkephalin) one of two naturally occurring substances in the brain which are neurotransmitters and have an opiate like effect, suppressing the sensation of pain.

encephalitis inflammation of the brain tissue.

encephalocele hernia of the brain tissue through a congenital or traumatic opening in the skull.

endemic describes an infectious disease which is always present to a lesser or greater degree in a particular locality.

endo- combining form meaning within or inner.

endocervical pertaining to the endocervix.

endocervicitis inflammation of the epithelium and glands within the cervix.

endocervix the glandular mucous membrane lining the uterine cervix.

endocrine system glands which secrete their produce, mainly hormones, directly into the bloodstream.

endoderm the innermost of the three layers forming the embryonic disc which will form the cavities, passages and internal organs of the developing fetus.

endogenous produced from within (*compare* exogenous).

endometrial referring to the inner layer or mucous membrane lining the cavity of the uterus.

endometrial hyperplasia an overgrowth of the endometrial lining resulting from oestrogen stimulation without the controlling effect of progesterone.

endometrial polyp an overgrowth of endometrium which has formed on a stalk; it may protrude through the cervix. Usually benign but may cause abnormal bleeding.

endometriosis presence of functional endometrial tissue in abnormal locations, outside of the uterus.

endometrium the mucous membrane lining the inside of the body of the uterine cavity.

endorphins a number of different neuropeptides which act on the central nervous system and reduce the sensation of pain.

endotoxins poisonous substances released from the cell walls of micro-organisms. *Endotoxic shock* is a sudden physical collapse associated with septicaemia.

endotracheal tube a patent tube inserted via the nose or mouth into the trachea to maintain the airway during anaesthesia. A cuff around its base is inflated to ensure a good fit and prevent material or fluid passing down beside the tube into the lungs. Its use prevents Mendelson's syndrome during induction of general anaesthesia in pregnant women.

enema introduction of fluid into the rectum for therapeutic purposes.

engagement entry of the presenting part of the fetus into the true pelvis such that the widest part is below the brim.

engorgement a state of being overfilled. Engorgement of the breasts may occur as milk 'comes in' during lactation.

enteric referring to the intestines.

enteritis inflammation of the intestinal mucosa.

entoderm the innermost of the three primary germ layers of the inner cell mass which will become the internal organs of the fetus.

Entonox® an analgesic preparation consisting of premixed gases – 50% nitrous oxide and 50% oxygen. Inhaled during labour contractions to dull the pain sensation.

environmental health the totality of the various substances, gases, forces and attitudes in and about a community which affect the health of members of that community.

enzyme a substance capable of breaking down another substance by a chemical reaction.

eosin a red acid dye used in histopathology for staining bacteria or cells.

eosinophil a white granulocytic cell whose granules stain red with eosin.

epidemic an outbreak of a specific disease extending throughout a local community.

epidermal naevus (naevus verrocosus) a brown, warty lesion on the discoloured skin of the newborn caused by an overgrowth of epidermis.

epidermis the top or superficial layer of the skin.

epidermolysis bullosa a hereditary skin condition characterized by widespread development of vesicles on contact, without the occurrence of trauma.

epididymis the tightly coiled single duct into which spermatozoa are deposited and reach complete maturation before passing into the vas deferens.

epidural situated over the dura mater.

epidural analgesia pain relief achieved by introduction of local analgesia into the epidural space.

epidural blood patch treatment employed in the management of a dural puncture sustained during epidural catheterization. A small volume of the woman's blood is injected into the dural space; the clot which forms seals the breach and prevents further leakage of cerebrospinal fluid.

epigastric pertaining to the upper middle section of the abdomen.

epigastric pain pain in the upper area of the abdomen. May be a sign (with other indications) of an impending eclamptic fit.

epigastric region the upper middle part of the abdomen.

epilepsy recurring episodes of neurological malfunction including motor and sensory lapses or convulsive seizures and unconsciousness.

episiorraphy repair of an episiotomy.

episiotomy an incision made in the pelvic floor during childbirth to enlarge the vaginal orifice (*see* Figure 47).

epispadias a congenital defect in which the urethral canal opens on the underside of the penis.

epistaxis nosebleed.

epithelium a tissue compound identified by shape and function lining all inner body surfaces.

epoprostenol (prostacyclin) (PG1) one of the prostaglandin hormones. It is metabolized in vascular walls and inhibits platelet aggregation.

Epstein's pearls small white spots found on both sides of the hard palate in the mouth of a newborn baby.

Erb's palsy upper brachial plexus nerve damage resulting in paralysis of the upper arm.

erectile capable of becoming firm or dilated.

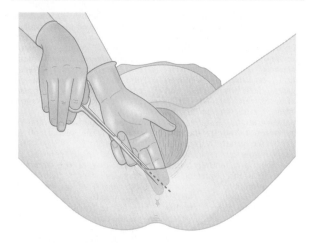

■ **Figure 47** Episiotomy

erectile tissue spongy tissue which, as a result of venous engorgement, becomes rigid and enlarged (*see* Figure 48). The penis and the nipple both contain erectile tissue.

ergometrine an oxytocic drug used prophylactically at the end of labour for the prevention or control of haemorrhage. It works by causing strong sustained contraction of smooth muscles, especially the uterus.

ergot a fungus developed on rye, the alkaloids of which are used in the manufacture of oxytocins.

erosion of the cervix destruction of superficial squamous epithelium and exposure of columnar epithelial cells of the endocervix.

erythema patchy redness of the skin.

erythema neonatorum patchy redness of variable size and shape on the body of a neonate. May be caused by heat, irritants or drugs but usually disappears after several days.

erythroblast an immature erythrocyte in which a nucleus is present.

erythroblastosis fetalis a haemolytic anaemia in the neonate resulting from maternal–fetal blood group incompatibility. The mother may form antibodies to the fetus's foreign antigen where it is of a differing Rh factor or ABO blood group.

erythrocyte a mature nonnucleated red cell able to transport oxygen around the body.

erythropoiesis the process by which red blood cells are formed.

Escherichia coli *see* E. coli.

estimated date of birth (EDB) a projected guess of the date on which the baby will be born; only 3–4% of babies are born on the date calculated. It is estimated using Nägele's rule, and calculations may be adjusted to take into account personal factors such as menstrual history.

estimated date of delivery (EDD) *see* estimated date of birth.

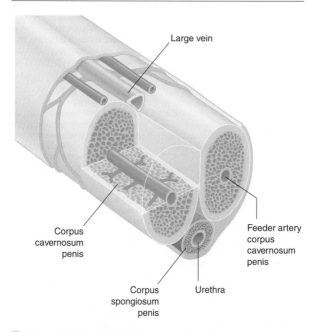

Large vein

Corpus
cavernosum
penis

Feeder artery
corpus
cavernosum
penis

Corpus
spongiosum
penis

Urethra

■ **Figure 48** Erectile tissue

estradiol, estriol *see* oestrogen.

estrone an oestrogen which can be isolated in the urine during pregnancy.

ethnic group a social group with shared values, beliefs, history and sometimes religion.

ethnography the study of an aspect of the life of a single culture, race or group within society.

eugenics branch of science concerned with gene selection and improvement of stock.

eutocia normal childbirth and labour.

evacuation emptying of the contents of e.g. uterus or bowel.

evaluate assess the value or worth of something, e.g. research results, care management, etc.

evidence statement or facts used as proof.

evidence based learning (EBL) also known as inquiry based learning (IBL) or problem based learning (PBL). A programme or course of study designed to enable students to participate in their own learning by exploring different types of evidence and knowledge. An educationalist oversees the process. Some student midwives' training is based wholly or in part on this system.

ex- combining form meaning outside, out of.

exacerbation an increase in the severity of a disease; making worse.

exchange   transfusion a methodical   and   gradual

withdrawal of almost all of a person's volume of blood and replacement with that provided by a donor. Can be done for neonates with severe jaundice and rhesus incompatibility.

excision the cutting away of a part of an organ or tissue.

excreta waste materials which have been removed from the body.

exercise physical activity or training to sustain or improve health.

exogenous originating from an external source (*compare* endogenous).

exomphalos a herniation of abdominal content into the umbilicus. It may or may not be covered with skin.

experiment an investigation in which one or more factors in a situation may be examined, altered and the effects studied; procedures used for testing a hypothesis.

expert witness a person with a great deal of experience and knowledge in a particular area who is able to testify or give evidence in a court of law.

expertise special skill in, knowledge of a particular area.

expulsion the act of forcing out, e.g. a fetus from the uterus.

expulsive stage of labour the period in labour after full dilation of the cervix during which the mother feels an overwhelming urge to use her abdominal muscles to push the fetus through the birth canal.

exsanguinate to empty of blood. This can happen to a fetus if the umbilical cord ruptures.

extended family the cousins, aunts, grandparents and significant others in a tightly knit group living in a large household or in close proximity to each other.

extension an action by which a flexed part is straightened out, e.g. the fetal head.

external ballottement bimanual examination in which an organ is tapped in an attempt to displace its contents which rebound and settle against the examiner's hand (*see* Figure 12, above).

external fertilization the sperm and ovum fuse outside the body of the mother, for example in a laboratory, as in in vitro fertilization (IVF).

external os uteri the opening in the cervix nearest the outside.

external version transabdominal manipulation of the fetus by which the lie or presentation is altered.

extrauterine outside the uterine cavity.

extrauterine pregnancy one that occurs outside of the uterus, as in an ectopic or an abdominal pregnancy.

extravasation leakage of body fluids out of the appropriate place or into surrounding tissues.

extrophy malformation of an organ.

exudates fluids such as sweat or protein rich substances and cells which leak out of the body through pores or pass through vessel walls into adjacent tissue.

Ff

F abbreviation for Fahrenheit, a scale of temperature measurement in which water freezes at 32°F and boiling point is 212°F.

face anterior part of the head extending from the forehead to chin. In the fetus it is the area between the supraorbital ridges and the mentum.

face presentation an extended cephalic presentation of the fetus. The face will be felt on vaginal examination.

face delivery occurs when there is a cephalic presentation of the fetus, but with the occiput occupying the hollow of the sacrum. The baby's face is born facing upwards towards the mother's face rather than facing backwards towards her spine, as in the birth of an anteriorly-positioned baby (*see* Figure 49).

face-to-pubes delivery occurs with a cephalic presentation, usually when the head is not fully flexed and has passed through the pelvis in an occipitoposterior position. As crowning occurs the brow will be seen under the symphysis pubis. The occipit sweeps (stretches excessively and tears) the perineum as it is born by flexion. It will probably be born before the face has completely emerged from under the symphysis pubis.

facial palsy damage to the 7th cranial nerve resulting in

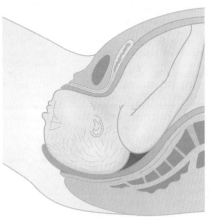

Face presentation
MA

■ **Figure 49** Face delivery

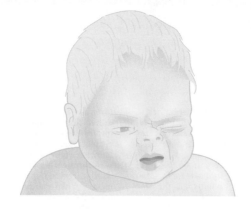

■ **Figure 50** Facial palsy

partial or total weakness of the muscles of expression (*see* Figure 50). Occasionally occurs as a result of a forceps delivery.

facilitator a person who enables or encourages another person to explore or discover information they need to fulfil their needs. A midwife during parentcraft classes will act as a facilitator for parents' enquiries.

factor a substance which promotes or enables a particular physiologic function.

Factors I, II, III, IV, V, VI, VII, VIII, IX, X, XI, XII, XIII names given to substances which enable blood to clot.

faeces food residue expelled as waste material from the bowels.

failed forceps unsuccessful attempt at delivery of the fetal head using obstetric forceps. An emergency caesarean section may be required.

failure to thrive deficit in the expected development of the infant. The neonate does not gain weight or meet the expected milestones.

faint sudden lapse of consciousness resulting from a fall in blood pressure and cerebral hypoxia.

fallectomy surgical removal of one or both fallopian tubes.

fallopian tubes the two oviducts or uterine tubes extending from the cornea and branching out to surround the ovary.

Fallot's tetralogy four congenital heart defects occurring together.

false labour discomfort or pain caused by uterine contractions but not resulting in cervical dilation.

false negative an incorrect diagnostic result indicating the absence of a pathological state when a disease is actually present.

false pelvis the region of the pelvis above the iliopectineal line.

false positive an incorrect diagnostic result suggesting that there is an abnormality when there is not.

falx a sickle-shaped structure.

falx cerebelli the sickle-shaped membrane of dura mater attached to the occipital bone and located between the two cerebral hemispheres.

falx cerebri the sickle-shaped, double-fold dura mater separating the two cerebral hemispheres.

familial pertaining to or occurring among family members.

family a group of people descended from a common ancestor; parents and children.

family planning premeditated measures adopted for limiting or timing the spacing of the birth of children.

Farber test microscopic examination of the meconium to detect lanugo, cells and ingested substances, the absence of which suggests intestinal obstruction.

fascia the fibrous sheath of connective tissue between muscles or loosely applied around organs, nerves and blood vessels.

fasting abstaining from food (but not water).

fasting blood sugars a glucose challenge test in which the body's response to a glucose load is compared to that of known healthy subjects. There should be an initial rise but a return to normal levels within 2 hours. Persistent elevation is associated with diabetes.

fatal resulting in death.

fear emotion based on anxiety and acute sense of alarm associated with an event or object.

fear–tension–pain syndrome a related phenomenological cycle first described by Grantly Dick Read as intensifying the pain of labour.

febrile characterized by fever.

fecundation the process of fertilization.

fecundity the ability to procreate.

feed to provide with nutrition; to give food to an infant by breast, bottle, tube or other means.

feeling the capacity to experience a sensation causing emotion.

female circumcision excision of various parts of the female genitalia for non-therapeutic reasons. This practice is illegal in the UK.

female genital mutilation female circumcision; removal of all or part of the labia minora, clitoris and labia majora.

female pseudohermaphrodite congenital abnormality of the external genitalia where the gender cannot be determined by examination of the external characteristics but ovaries are present.

feminism the promotion of women's rights to be equal to those of men.

femoral pertaining to the femur or thigh bone.

Ferguson's reflex the uncontrollable desire to bear down and aid expulsion of the fetus, triggered by pressure from the presenting part stimulating nerves in the pelvic floor.

fern test the pattern created by dried crystallized cervical mucus on a glass slide post ovulation. Indicative of the presence of an oestrogen surge.

ferritin an iron–protein complex. A form of iron stored in tissues.

fertile able to produce offspring.

fertile period the days in the menstrual cycle after ovulation during which a pregnancy is likely to occur.

fertility rate the number of births per 1000 women.

fertilization the union of male and female gametes (*see* Figure 51).

fetal pertaining to the fetus.

fetal alcohol syndrome a collection of abnormalities,

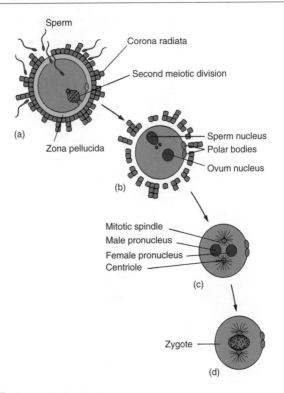

Figure 51 Fertilization

including facial abnormalities, mental retardation and small-ness for gestational age, seen in infants whose mothers have consumed large quantities of alcohol in pregnancy.

fetal blood sampling procedure performed in labour, whereby a small sample of blood is obtained from the scalp of the fetus for estimation of pH and blood gases as a means of determining fetal well-being (*see* Figure 52).

fetal bradycardia a slow fetal heart rate of less than 100 beats per minute (normal = 110–150 b.p.m.).

fetal circulation the cardio-vascular network in the fetus including the placenta and umbilical cord (*see* Figure 53).

fetal death the fetus dies in utero before the onset of labour.

fetal distress usually indicated by loss of beat-to-beat varia-tion, bradycardia, tachycardia or late decelerations.

fetal haemoglobin HbF, the dominant haemoglobin in intrauterine life, though small

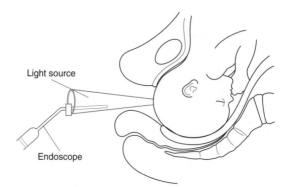

Light source

Endoscope

■ **Figure 52** Fetal blood sampling

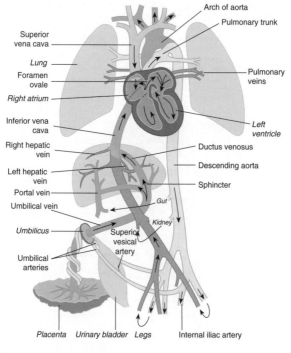

Arch of aorta

Pulmonary trunk

Superior vena cava

Lung

Foramen ovale

Right atrium

Pulmonary veins

Inferior vena cava

Left ventricle

Right hepatic vein

Ductus venosus

Left hepatic vein

Descending aorta

Portal vein

Sphincter

Umbilical vein

Gut

Umbilicus

Kidney

Superior vesical artery

Umbilical arteries

Placenta   *Urinary bladder*   *Legs*

Internal iliac artery

■ **Figure 53** Fetal circulation

quantities continue to be produced throughout life. It is highly receptive to oxygen but is fragile and therefore short-lived.

fetal heart rate (FHR) the number of times the fetal heart beats in 1 minute – normal range is between 110 and 150 beats per minute.

fetal heart sounds the sound of the fetal heart beat which can be auscultated and counted.

fetal hypoxia a state of reduced delivery of oxygen to the fetus.

fetal movements movements made by the fetus in utero. These are present from the beginning of pregnancy but cannot be felt by the mother before the 16th to 19th week of gestation. Normally, the mother should feel at least 10 movements in a 12-hour period.

fetal skull the entire bony structure of the fetal head including the three regions of face, vault and base.

feticide the destruction or killing of a fetus in utero.

fetology the study of the fetus in utero.

fetoplacental referring to the fetus and placenta to which it is attached as one unit/organism.

fetoscopy transabdominal introduction of an instrument into the uterine cavity for visual inspection of the fetus.

fetus term applied to mammalian offspring from the beginning of the 9th week after fertilization until birth.

fetus papyraceous one of twin fetuses that has died early in pregnancy and has been flattened by the survivor to resemble a paper cutout.

fetus sanguinolentis a fetus that has died and started to decompose and is born with dark blood patches visible beneath the skin.

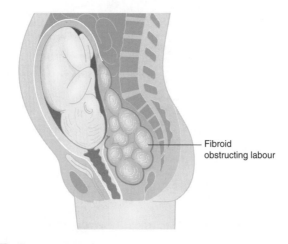

Fibroid obstructing labour

■ **Figure 54** Fibroid

fever a rise in body temperature above normal limits.

fibrin an insoluble protein formed by the interaction of thrombin and fibrinogen during clot formation.

fibrinogen the soluble protein precursor of fibrin present in blood plasma.

fibrinolysin the enzyme in the blood which dissolves fibrin.

fibroid a dense mass of adherent fibrous tissue (*see* Figure 54). A benign tumour found within the muscle of the uterus.

fibromyoma a benign tumour of uterine muscle; a fibroid.

fibromyomectomy surgical removal of a fibroid.

fight or flight reaction a state of heightened preparedness for sudden activity resulting from a surge of adrenaline (epinephrine) in the circulation as a consequence of great stress. Larger amounts of energy become available and peripheral circulation is depleted. It is counterproductive in labour.

filter a porous membrane-like structure which permits selective passage of some compounds while restricting the passage of others.

filtrate the solution that has passed through a filter.

fimbria 1. a fringe. 2. the fringe-like dilated extremity of the fallopian tube.

fimbria ovarica the fringe or fringe-like end of the fallopian tube which is nearest to the ovary.

first degree tear laceration of the perineum involving only the skin or fourchette.

first stage of labour the interval from the onset of labour to complete dilation of the cervix (*see* Figure 55).

fission 1. cleavage or splitting. 2. a method of asexual reproduction.

fissure 1. groove or cleft normally occurring in the body. 2. ulceration or crack in the skin.

fistula abnormal communication between two surfaces or organs.

fit a convulsion or seizure.

flaccid relaxed or without tone; soft, flabby, limp.

flagellum (PLURAL flagella) thin, whip-like process contained in cytoplasm, movement of which enables propulsion in certain bacteria and sperm cells.

Flagyl® trade name for the antimicrobial drug metronidazole.

flank the side abdominal region between the ribs and hip.

flaring of nostrils dilation of the nares (nostrils) to aid respiratory effort where breathing is difficult, e.g. in respiratory distress syndrome in a preterm neonate.

flat pelvis (SYNONYM platypelloid pelvis) a pelvis with reduced anteroposterior and increased transverse diameters and a shallow cavity.

flatulence an excess of gas in the stomach or intestines.

fleshy mole *see* carneous mole.

flexion the state of being bent. The normal attitude or position of the fetal head in relation to its body in utero.

flooding term used to describe heavy menstrual blood flow.

flora bacteria found in the large intestine which enable the body to manufacture essential vitamins such as vitamin K and protect against invasion by pathological organisms.

fluid balance the maintenance of optimal water content for physiologic function by regulating intake and output.

fluid overload excessive accumulation of fluid within the body as a result of overtransfusion of intravenous solutions.

fluid thrill a clinical sign indicative of polyhydramnios. A

Second stage = FETAL EXPULSION
From full dilatation
➝ birth of baby

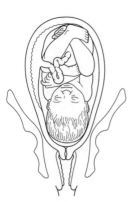

Third stage
From birth of baby ➝ expulsion
of placenta and membranes
(and uterus retracted firmly)

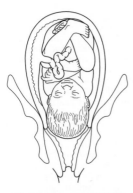

First stage = DILATATION
From onset of regular uterine
contractions and effacement of
cervix and dilatation of os
➝ full dilatation of os uteri

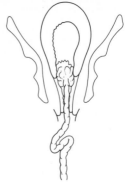

■ **Figure 55** Stages of labour

ripple or wave effect can be seen over the abdomen when one side is tapped.

Foley catheter a balloon-tipped retainable urinary catheter.

folic acid a vitamin of the B complex group found in green leafy vegetables, liver and yeast; essential to the development of healthy erythrocytes.

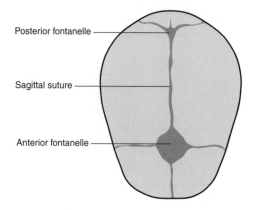

Posterior fontanelle

Sagittal suture

Anterior fontanelle

■ **Figure 56** Fontanelle

follicle a small secretory sac or cavity.

follicle stimulating hormone (FSH) pituitary hormone which stimulates growth and maturation of ovarian follicles or spermatogenesis in the testes.

follicular phase the early period of the menstrual cycle during which the graafian follicle is growing and ripening.

fontanelle a membranous space between the cranial bones in the fetus and neonate (*see* Figure 56).

footling presentation a variation of the breech presentation in which one foot is presenting in front of the buttocks.

foramen an opening or perforation, especially in a bone.

foramen magnum the large opening at the base of the skull through which the spinal cord passes.

foramen ovale oval window; a physiological opening in the septum of the heart through which blood is shunted from the right to left atrium in fetal life, bypassing the lungs.

forceps a two-bladed surgical instrument used to grasp or compress body tissues or objects.

forceps delivery an assisted birth in which extraction of the fetus is enabled by the application of forceps to the head and traction (*see* Figure 57).

forceps rotation use of Kielland's rotational forceps which have long handles and flat or less defined curvatures of the blade to correct malposition of the fetal head.

foremilk the first milk drawn at each breastfeed.

foreskin (SYNONYM prepuce) the skin covering the glans penis.

forewaters the pool of amniotic fluid lying in front of the presenting part and separated from the main volume (*see* Figure 58).

formaldehyde a powerful disinfectant.

formula 1. rules expressed in symbols. 2. laboratory-prepared recipe of modified cows' milk for feeding infants.

fornication 1. sexual intercourse. 2. historically, sexual intercourse outside marriage.

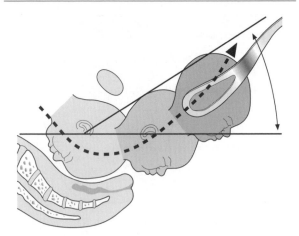

■ Figure 57 Forceps delivery

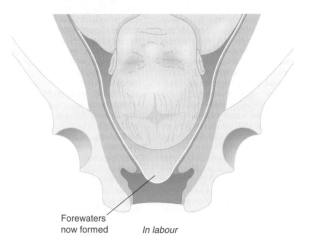

Forewaters
now formed   *In labour*

■ Figure 58 Forewaters

fornix 1. a cul-de-sac or arch-shaped structure. 2. the recessed arched vault of the vagina between the cervix and the vaginal walls (*see* Figure 59).

Fortral® (pentazocine) moderate to strong analgesic drug which may be given in early labour.

fossa a depression or hollow.

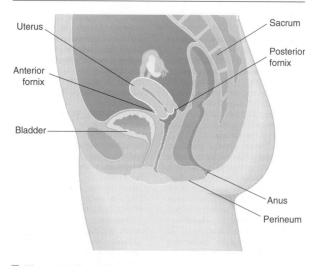

Uterus

Sacrum

Posterior fornix

Anterior fornix

Bladder

Anus

Perineum

■ **Figure 59** Fornix

Foundation for the Study of Infant Deaths (FSID) a charity which raises funds to carry out research and offer support to bereaved parents.

fourchette a fold of skin at the posterior aspect of the labia minora.

fracture break of a bone or cartilage.

fracture of the clavicle a break in the long bone lying between the shoulder girdle and the sternum. It may be deliberately broken (cleidotomy) to release the baby's shoulder in cases of shoulder dystocia.

fracture of the skull a break in one of the bones of the skull. May occur following a forceps delivery.

frank extended breech the fetus is presenting with the buttocks over the cervical os, the thighs are flexed and the legs are extended to lie alongside the shoulders.

frenulum a small fold of mucous membrane acting as a restraining ligament.

frenulum of the tongue the membranous cord which attaches the tongue to the floor of the mouth.

friable easily broken or torn, crumbly.

Friedman's curve a curved line on pre-printed partograms which indicates the expected progress of labour (by medical definitions). If the woman's progress does not parallel the curve and deviates to the right by more than 2 hours, augmentation of labour may be offered.

frigid term used to describe a woman who does not experience sexual arousal or enjoy sexual intercourse.

frontal pertaining to the anterior aspect of the body or the forehead.

FSH *see* follicle stimulating hormone.

full term a term used to describe a woman who has reached 37 completed weeks of pregnancy or beyond.

fulminating sudden, severe and rapid in onset or progression.

fulminating pre-eclampsia condition in which a client with pre-eclampsia is at risk of experiencing a seizure.

fundal referring to the fundus, or top of the uterus.

fundal force (fundal pressure) the application of force to the top of the uterus to aid delivery of the infant in the second stage of labour or the placenta in the third stage. Not generally considered safe in current practice, except in emergency situations.

fundal height estimation of the gestational age by measuring the distance from the top of the uterus to the symphysis pubis.

fundal placenta a placenta normally located in the top or fundus of the uterus.

fundus the base of an organ or the part farthest removed from the opening.

fungal infection pathogenic condition caused by a fungus or yeast.

funic referring to the umbilical cord (funis).

funic souffle a soft blowing murmur emitted from the umbilical cord and usually synchronous with beating of the fetal heart.

funnel pelvis a pelvis in which there is progressive reduction of the diameters from the brim to outlet.

fusion joining together, e.g. of organs, cavities or tubes. Dividing walls are removed by ingestion by enzymes.

Gg

g (gm) abbreviation for gram.

gag 1. to retch. 2. an instrument used to prevent closure of the jaw.

gag reflex constriction of the pharyngeal muscle in response to stimulation of the soft palette, the tongue is pulled back to protect the airway.

G6PD *see* glucose-6-phosphate dehydrogenase.

gait a manner of walking or carrying one's body.

galactagogue an agent that increases the secretion of milk.

galacto-, galact combining form denoting milk.

galactorrhoea lactation not associated with childbirth.

galactosaemia inability to convert galactose to glucose. Caused by an inborn error of metabolism in which the galactose splitting enzyme galactose-1-phosphate uridyl transferase is either deficient or absent.

galactose a monosaccharide produced after the metabolism of lactose.

galactosis secretion of milk by the mammary glands.

Galant reflex induced sidewards flexion of the neonate's hips in the direction of contact when the lower back is stroked.

Galen's vein (vein of Galen) the large cerebral vein which drains blood from the mid-brain. During abnormal moulding or a difficult delivery it may rupture causing severe intracranial haemorrhage.

gall bile.

gall bladder a hollow, pear-shaped structure situated on the undersurface of the liver in which bile is stored and concentrated.

gamete the reproductive cells capable of fertilization.

gamete intrafallopian transfer (GIFT) ovum and sperm are collected, fertilized in a test tube and then implanted into the uterus.

gametocyte a cell which has the potential to become a sperm or ovum.

gametogenesis the process of formation and development of gametes.

gametophyte a stage in the process of gamete development at which the nuclei are haploid.

gamma globulin a group of immunoglobulins, A, D, E, G and M, with specific antibody activity.

ganglion a body of nerve cells from which other fibres or tendrils extend.

gangrene tissue death and necrosis due to failure or interruption of blood supply.

Gardnerella vaginalis a rod shaped gram-negative bacterium normally found in the vagina. *Gardnerella vaginalis vaginitis* is the inflammation and symptoms resulting from bacterial infection with *Gardnerella*; thought to be transmitted sexually.

gas matter in vaporous state, being neither solid nor liquid.

gastric juices secretions of the glands in the stomach; these are strongly acid and digest food.

gastric lavage washing out of the stomach.

gastric tube feeding introduction of food into the stomach via a tube. A method often employed in the care of premature or sick babies.

gastro- combining form meaning pertaining to the stomach.

gastroenteritis inflammation of the stomach and intestinal mucosa; usually accompanied by vomiting and diarrhoea.

gate control theory of pain suggests that there is selection or competition as to which impulses will travel up the spine and be received in the brain, for example sensations such as electricity across the skin or pain from contraction compete. When TENS (transcutaneous electrical nerve stimulation) is used, electricity, rather than pain, passes up the spinal nerves (*see* Figure 99).

gel a thick substance with a high concentration of water used as a lubricant or to deliver medicine.

gender the classification of people as female or male.

gene a unit of hereditary factor capable of transmitting specific genetic code and occupying a defined position on a chromosome.

gene pool the total number of genetic traits available within a population.

general anaesthesia a drug-induced medical state in which there is combined loss of sensation and consciousness.

general practitioner a doctor engaged in primary practice within the community; accessible by client made appointment.

generation all people considered to be within a specific age band; the time between the birth of an individual and the birth of his/her offspring.

genetic pertaining to genes; having reference to the origin of development.

genetic carrier a person who carries a 'faulty' gene which can be passed on to his or her children but who displays no signs of it or of ill health.

genetic counselling detailed explanation of the risks of transmitting a hereditary condition to one's children and presentation of options or reproductive alternatives.

genetic engineering manipulation of genetic characteristics by removal or insertion of foreign gene materials.

genetic screening DNA analysis of blood samples to determine which characteristic an offspring is likely to inherit.

genetics the study of heredity.

genital relating to the organs of reproduction.

genital wart small, cauliflower-like swellings on the vulva or prepuce caused by a virus. These may spread during pregnancy.

genitalia the organs of reproduction.

genitourinary relating to the function of the urinary and genital organs.

genome map pictorial representation showing the location of the genes on each chromosome.

genotype mapping of the individual genetic make-up.

genupectoral position resting upon the knees and chest, with head down and hips elevated.

genus a classification of plants or animals by family or species grouping.

germ a common term applied to any micro-organism. A substance, protoplasm, seed or spore capable of development into a new individual or whole organism.

German measles *see* rubella.

germicide an agent that kills germs.

gestation process of being carried or carrying in the womb; pregnancy.

gestational age the duration of the pregnancy indicates the likely maturity of the fetus, usually calculated from the first day of the last menstrual period.

gestational diabetes diabetes arising in the second half of pregnancy with spontaneous resolution after delivery. The problems associated with diabetes may occur.

gigantism abnormally large stature.

gingivitis inflammation of the mucous membranes and underlying soft tissues of the gum.

girdle a structure or band which encircles the body. The *pelvic girdle* is the bony encircling structure formed by the two innominate bones and the sacrum.

glabella the bony prominence formed by the joining of the frontal bones and supraorbital ridges.

gland a collection of tissue or specialized cells capable of secreting and excreting materials used to influence other bodily functions.

glans of clitoris erectile tissue at the end of the clitoris.

glans penis the expanded tip of the penis.

globin one of a class of proteins obtained from haemoglobin.

globulin a large group of plasma proteins; alpha, beta and gamma, that are characterized by their solubility in dilute salt solutions.

glomerulus a small rounded mass; the microscopic loops of capillaries, millions of which make up the kidney.

glossitis inflammation of the tongue.

glucagon hormones produced in the islets of Langerhans that stimulate conversion of glycogen to glucose.

glucose crystalline monosaccharide, dextrose, obtained by the incomplete hydrolysis of carbohydrates.

glucose-6-phosphate dehydrogenase (G6PD) an enzyme found in erythrocytes and other cells; a deficiency of this enzyme may trigger spontaneous haemolysis and ensuing jaundice.

glucose tolerance test (GTT) a diagnostic test for diabetes. The person is given a strong glucose drink and blood is taken every half-hour for several hours to monitor the level of blood glucose and how the body deals with it.

glucosuria presence of glucose in the urine.

glucuronyl transferase a liver enzyme that hydrolyzes fat-soluble bilirubin to an easily excreted water-soluble form.

gluteal pertaining to the buttocks or region of the buttocks.

gluteal muscle the largest muscle group in the buttocks.

glycerin a sweet, colourless fluid obtained from hydrolized fats; used to carry medicine, moisten skin and lips and soften stools.

glycogen energy source formed from carbohydrates which are stored in the liver and muscles and converted into glucose when needed.

glycogenesis the formation of glycogen.

glycogenolysis the process of breaking down and liberation of glucagon from the liver to other tissues.

glycosuria presence of sugar in the urine.

gnath-, gnatho- combining form denoting the jaw.

goitre swelling of the front of the neck caused by enlargement of the thyroid gland.

gonadotrophic hormone a hormone which stimulates activity in the gonads.

gonads a general term for glands or organs producing gametes; the testicles and ovaries.

gonococcus (PLURAL gono-cocci) the organism causing gonorrhoea, *Neisseria gonorrhoeae.*

gonorrhoea an easily treated sexually transmitted disease. If untreated, contact with the discharge during vaginal birth may cause ophthalmia neonatorum and blindness in the neonate.

graafian follicle the cystic structure surrounding the mature ovum on the surface of the ovary which secretes oestrogen (*see* Figure 60).

gram staining a laboratory technique used to classify bacteria; having been exposed to alcohol, they either take up a staining lotion (*gram-positive*) or do not (*gram-negative*).

grand multipara defining term for a woman of high parity, having given birth to more than four children.

granulation an upward migration of newly formed capillaries and fibroblasts seen in wound healing.

granulosa cells epithelial cells lining the graafian follicle.

grasp reflex the primitive reflex which can be triggered in the neonate by stroking the palm of the hands or sole of the foot. The fingers will curl around the stimulator and the resultant grasp is so strong as to enable the infant to be lifted.

gravid pregnant.

gravida a pregnant woman.

gravidum gingivitis inflammation of the mucous membrane and underlying tissues of the

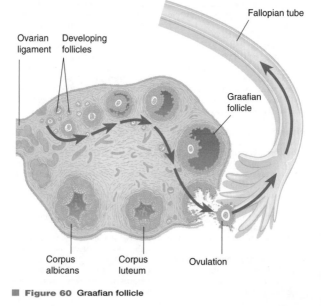

Fallopian tube

Ovarian ligament

Developing follicles

Graafian follicle

Corpus albicans

Corpus luteum

Ovulation

■ **Figure 60 Graafian follicle**

gum; associated with pregnancy hormones.

grief physical manifestation of bereavement, separation or loss of a person or object with whom there is an emotional attachment.

groin the depressed region between the abdomen and thighs.

gross large enough to be seen without magnification.

group practice an establishment where several practitioners work together.

growth hormone a hormone directly influencing carbohydrate, fat and protein metabolism and promoting growth.

growth retardation failure of expected progress in growth in a fetus or neonate.

grunting abnormal respiratory sound noted on expiration indicating that the glottis has closed to the flow of air out of the lung, usually to prevent collapse of the lung. Heard in preterm infants suffering from respiratory distress syndrome.

gumma a lesion of tertiary syphilis.

gut the intestine; the embryonic digestive tract consists of foregut, midgut and hindgut.

Guthrie test a screening test to diagnose phenylketonuria. Often used as a generic term to include the other tests carried out at the same time

gyn-, gynae, gyno- combining terms meaning woman.

gynaecoid woman-like; having female characteristics.

gynaecoid pelvis pelvis, the size and shape of which is ideal for childbirth.

gynaecology a branch of medicine devoted to treating diseases of women, especially conditions of the reproductive organs and genitalia.

Hh

H symbol for hydrogen.

habitual abortion more than three consecutive abortions.

haem-, haemo- combining form denoting blood.

haemangioma a non-cancerous tumour composed of a mass of blood vessels.

haematemesis vomiting of blood.

haematocele collection of blood in a cavity.

haematocrit the percentage of whole blood occupied by red cells.

haematology the scientific study of the nature of blood, its function and diseases.

haematoma a mass formed by a collection of blood (*see* Figure 61).

haematometra a collection of blood or menstrual fluid in the uterus.

haematosalpinx a collection of blood in the fallopian tube.

haematuria presence of blood in the urine.

haemoconcentration reduction of the fluid volume in the bloodstream.

haemodialysis a process in which blood is drained from the body a little at a time, mechanically filtered to remove impurities and returned. May be required if renal failure follows a severe haemorrhage.

haemodilution increase in the ratio of plasma to cells in the bloodstream. Normal physiology of early pregnancy is accompanied by a lowering of the haemoglobin.

haemoglobin the respiratory property of erythrocytes, con-

sisting of four haem iron molecules linked to the protein globin and carrying out the dual functions of absorbing and releasing oxygen.

haemoglobin F normal haemoglobin of the fetus, more fragile than adult haemoglobin and capable of absorbing oxygen at a lower tension.

haemolysin a substance which frees haemoglobin from red cells.

haemolysis the destruction of red cells and liberation of haemoglobin.

haemolytic having the ability to cause haemolysis.

haemolytic jaundice jaundice resulting from the destruction of excessive haemoglobin not required in extrauterine life. The resulting bile pigments remain in the circulation causing a yellow discoloration to the skin, until they can be removed by the maturing liver.

haemophilia a sex-linked recessive inherited disease of delayed clotting, carried by females but manifesting in males.

Haemophilus a genus of bacteria dependent on blood pigments for growth.

haemopoiesis (SYNONYM haematopoiesis) the process of formation of blood.

haemoptysis coughing up of blood.

haemorrhage excessive loss of blood through injury or tissue damage. Can occur from the placental site in pregnancy, during the first, second or third stages of labour or in the early postnatal period. Serious

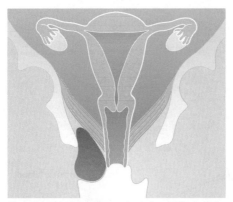

Haematoma in the perineum due to trauma lower in the genital tract or a vessel not being ligated during repair of the perineum

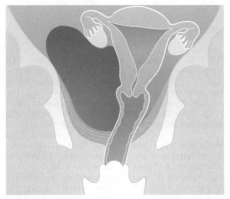

Concealed haematoma due to trauma high in the genital tract

■ **Figure 61** Haematoma

haemorrhage would be considered an obstetric emergency.

haemorrhagic diathesis an abnormal bleeding tendency as in haemophilia, vitamin K deficiency or disseminated intravascular coagulation.

haemorrhagic disease of the newborn bleeding tendency in the newborn. Hypothetically linked to deficiency of vitamin K in the neonate.

haemorrhoids (SYNONYM piles) the occurrence of varicose veins in the lower rectum and anus.

haemostasis the arrest of bleeding or haemorrhage.

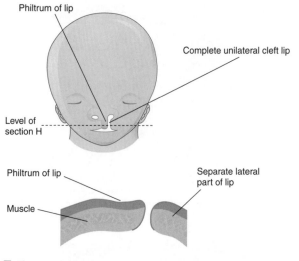

Philtrum of lip

Complete unilateral cleft lip

Level of section H

Philtrum of lip

Separate lateral part of lip

Muscle

■ **Figure 62** Hare lip

haemostatic a drug or agent that arrests bleeding or haemorrhage.

hallucination sensory stimulus (visual, aural, tactile, etc.) perceived by an individual but unconnected to events outside the body.

hand presentation when the hand lies lowest in the uterus in labour. This may occur when there is an uncorrected oblique lie allowing the arm and hand to prolapse into the vagina or as a compound presentation with the head.

handicap disability (e.g. hearing, vision, understanding) which causes a person to be less able in some area than an individual described as normal.

hard chancre a 'crusty' ulcerated lesion at the site of the primary syphilitic infection.

hard palate the anterior part of the roof of the mouth located behind the teeth.

hare lip old, colloquial term for cleft or clefts in the upper lip (*see* Figure 29 above, and Figure 62).

harlequin fetus a multi-coloured congenital skin condition. The infant's skin is covered in scaly patches with red fissures between them which crack, allowing seepage of serous fluid.

Hartmann's solution a fluid administered intravenously to expand the volume of the circulating plasma.

Hb abbreviation for haemoglobin.

HCG (human chorionic gonadotrophin) a water-soluble hormone produced by the trophoblast and excreted in the urine of pregnant women.

head box a five-sided perspex box with a cut-out section to fit around the infant's neck. It is put over the head of a sick baby to deliver higher concentrations of oxygen than are

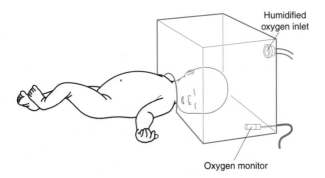

Humidified
oxygen inlet

Oxygen monitor

■ **Figure 63** Head box

available in the atmosphere (*see* Figure 63).

head fitting test an assessment made at term when there is non-engagement of the fetal head. An attempt is made to fit the non-engaged fetal head into the maternal pelvis thereby excluding cephalopelvic disproportion.

health authority the UK is divided into regional and local health authorities which are the administrative units of the National Health Service.

health care assistant a person who assists the professional person in simple tasks, sometimes of a domestic nature.

health education method employed to enable individuals or collective populations to adopt strategies aimed at improvement in health through change and prevention of disease.

health professional a person who has received some training in health care.

health visitor a person who is a registered nurse and a registered midwife (or who is trained in midwifery) and who has obtained additional post-registration qualification; health visitors work mainly with families and preschool children in primary care for the promotion of health.

heart the organ of circulation. A hollow muscular organ which functions as a pump maintaining circulation of the blood.

heart rate the speed at which the heart pumps blood around the body – normally 70–90 beats per minute (b.p.m.) in the adult and 110–150 in a fetus.

heartburn a burning sensation under the sternum caused by gastro-oesophageal reflux.

Hegar's dilators a set of surgical instruments of increasing size used to dilate the cervix from the outside inwards.

Hegar's sign a possible sign of early pregnancy – on bimanual palpation the softening of the uterus allows the fingers to nearly meet above the level of the cervix.

HELLP syndrome an acronym describing severe pregnancy-induced hypertension with complications – haemolysis, elevated liver enzymes, and low platelet levels.

hemicephalus condition where a fetus has only the lower

half of its brain tissue present.

hemiplegia paralysis of one side of the body.

heparin a naturally occurring protein which prevents intravascular clotting. It may be administered as preoperative preparation before caesarean section in high risk cases to prevent the formation of deep vein thrombosis.

hepatic pertaining to or involving the liver.

hepatitis inflammation of the liver. Can be caused by microorganisms, drugs, poisons or blood transfusions.

herbalist a therapist specializing in the medicinal properties of plants and who prescribes herbal infusions, tinctures, lotions and other preparations for medicinal use.

heredity the process by which traits, characteristics and diseases are passed from one generation to the next, on the chromosomes.

hermaphrodite an individual of indeterminable gender, possessing both male and female genital organs.

hernia the abnormal protrusion of an organ beyond or outside of its normal containing walls due to a weakness in the containing wall.

herpes an acute and highly contagious viral infection characterized by vesicle formation.

herpes genitalis an infectious viral infection causing painful oozing vesicular lesions on the mucous membranes of the vulva or penis.

herpes gestationis a generalized itching and vesicular rash accruing during the second and third trimester of pregnancy.

heterogenous different in kind or dissimilar.

heterotopic pregnancy a pregnancy occurring in an abnormal location, such as outside the uterine tubes or uterus.

heterozygous possessing dissimilar genes, for example a man whose blood group expression is rhesus positive, but who carries both positive and negative genes, and who is therefore able to father children that are either rhesus negative or rhesus positive.

Hg symbol for mercury, a liquid metal used in the manufacture of clinical thermometers.

hiatus an abnormal space or opening.

hiatus hernia a small protrusion of the stomach into the oesophageal hiatus.

high forceps forceps that are applied when the fetal head is high – more than 2 cm above the ischial spines.

high-risk infant an infant who is likely to suffer ill health or death.

high-risk pregnancy a pregnancy which may result in injury or death to the mother or fetus.

hind waters the amniotic fluid behind and trapped by the fetal head.

Hirschsprung's disease congenital abnormality caused by absence of ganglion cells in a section of the colon or rectum; characterized by spasm in the aganglionic region and distension proximal to the defect. It may result in constipation, acute abdominal distension and obstruction.

hirsute shaggy, hairy.

histamine a protein liberated when tissue is injured or comes into contact with a foreign agent. It triggers arterial spasm, erythema, capillary dilation with increased permeability and oedema.

histology a branch of biology dealing with the microscopic structure of tissues and cells of organs.

history taking obtaining a detailed account of the woman's family history, past and present medical, surgical and obstetric health on which to base future care.

HIV *see* human immunodeficiency virus.

holistic taking into account the whole, all aspects of the person/situation.

holoacardius acephalus the grossly abnormal twin of a normal fetus.

Homans' sign pain experienced in the calf and popliteal area on dorsiflexion of the foot. It is a positive sign of deep vein thrombosis.

home birth labour and birth in the home; may be planned or unplanned. For women whose pregnancies are uncomplicated, planned home birth is no less safe than hospital birth.

home confinement older, colloquial term for home birth.

homeopathy non-Western system of therapy often using herbs.

homeostasis the tendency to remain in a state of equilibrium or balance; the status quo; remaining stable, as it was.

homeothermic the ability of the body to maintain a stable temperature despite environmental conditions. This is not present in the neonate in the same way as an adult, which is why babies need to be kept warm.

homogeneous having the same qualities or being the same.

homologous chromosomes any two chromosomes that are identical in size and shape and carrying similar coding information in compatible sequence. Humans have 22 pairs and one different pair which denotes the gender of the individual.

homosexual 1. pertaining to the same sex. 2. a person who is attracted to people of the same sex.

homosexuality sexual attraction between people of the same sex.

homozygous having two genes which carry the same characteristic, e.g. a man who is homozygous rhesus positive carries two rhesus positive genes which means that he will always pass a rhesus positive gene on to any children he has.

hormones chemicals produced by endocrine glands and secreted into the bloodstream. They act to bring about specific regulatory effects on body parts remote from their origin.

hourglass constriction 1. an encircling contraction of an organ causing it to be divided more or less into two compartments. 2. contraction of the uterus occurring in the third stage of labour causing entrapment of the placenta; may be a cause of postpartum haemorrhage.

hourglass uterus an abnormal stricture occurring at the junction of the upper and lower uterine segment in which a band of circular muscles in the uterus contract independently causing lack of progress in labour.

Huhner's test fertility test carried out on seminal fluid withdrawn from the vaginal fornix 1 hour after intercourse. It is examined for sperm activity and survival.

human chorionic gonadotrophin (HCG) a hormone produced by the trophoblast after conception. Its action is to maintain the corpus luteum and prevent menstruation thereby ensuring the survival of the pregnancy.

human immunodeficiency virus (HIV) a slow-acting

retrovirus contained in blood and body fluids which destroys the immune system of the body. Main routes of transmission are unprotected penetrative sexual intercourse, blood transfusion, organ transplantation, vertically from mother to infant in utero or at birth or possibly through breastfeeding.

human placental lactogen (HPL) a growth-type hormone secreted by the placenta affecting carbohydrate metabolism.

humerus the bone of the upper arm.

Hutchinson's triad a term describing three linked indicators of congenital syphilis. The infant is born with interstitial keratitis, deafness, and will develop notched teeth.

hyaline a clear vitreous protein material found in various body tissues including the lungs.

hyaline membrane disease degeneration of the hyaline resulting in opacity.

hydatidiform mole degeneration of the placenta and proliferation of the trophoblast into hydropic vesicles resembling a bunch of grapes.

hydra-, hydro- combining form denoting water or hydrogen.

hydraemia a disproportionate increase in the volume of plasma to red cells in the blood.

hydralazine a hypotensive drug used in management of preeclampsia.

hydramnios normal volume of amniotic fluid.

hydration absorption of water.

hydrocele accumulation of fluid in the sac or tunica vaginalis of the testes. A common non-pathological condition in the neonate, which resolves spontaneously.

hydrocephalus enlargement of the head with water. A congenital defect caused by accumulation of cerebrospinal fluid, leading to distension of the ventricles and damage to the brain tissue.

hydrochloric acid a naturally occurring chemical component of gastric juices and essential to the digestion of food. Aspiration of hydrochloric acid into the lung causes Mendelson's syndrome.

hydrocortisone an adrenocortical steroid. May be given by injection to patients who are severely shocked.

hydrogen the lightest of the known gases which combines with oxygen to form water, H_2O.

hydrogen ions the positively electric charged nucleus. The pH of the blood is determined by the concentration of hydrogen ions.

hydronephrosis retention of urine with back pressure, dilation of the renal pelvis and destruction of the kidney substance secondary to obstruction.

hydrops fetalis severe and generalized oedema, jaundice and anaemia of the fetus due to rhesus incompatibility; may result in fetal death.

hydrops gravidarum oedema occurring in pregnancy.

hydrosalpinx fluid distension of the fallopian tubes.

hygiene 1. a group of practical approaches to attaining and maintaining health by preventing the multiplication of microorganisms. 2. the teaching of these approaches.

hygroma a cystic lymph-filled cavity occurring as a congenital malformation.

hymen a membranous structure partially blocking the orifice of the vagina before sexual intercourse.

hyoscine (scopolamine) drug used to depress the central nervous system which reduces salivary secretions and has amnesic properties.

hyper- combining term denoting excess or above normal.

hyperbilirubinaemia high blood levels of bilirubin, often seen in the neonate due to breakdown of red blood cells. Very high levels can cause kernicterus and brain damage.

hypercalcaemia excess of calcium in the circulation.

hypercapnia excess of carbon dioxide in the circulation.

hyperglycaemia excess of glucose in the circulation.

hyperemesis excessive vomiting.

hyperemesis gravidarum excessive vomiting in pregnancy. This can be a serious problem resulting in electrolyte imbalance.

hyperkalaemia excess of potassium in the circulation.

hyperlactation secretion of milk from the breasts beyond the normal duration of breastfeeding.

hypernatraemia excess of sodium in the circulation.

hyperphenylalaninaemia a positive indicator of the condition phenylketonuria in which there are high levels of the protein phenylalanine in the blood. If untreated it can lead to brain damage.

hyperplasia growth by increase in cell numbers.

hyperpyrexia a body temperature over 40°C.

hypersensitivity excess immunological response to a drug or allergen not experienced by the majority of people.

hypertension abnormally high blood pressure. Blood pressure is recorded in early pregnancy. If the diastolic blood pressure rises 20 mmHg above the recording in early pregnancy or above 90 mmHg diastolic the woman is said to have pregnancy-induced hypertension (PIH).

hyperthyroidism excessive secretion of thyroid hormones into the blood resulting in raised metabolic rate, hyperactivity, tachycardia, sweating, emaciation, tremor and exophthalmos.

hypertonia increase to excess in the tone or tension of muscles or blood vessels.

hypertonic solution a solution with an osmotic pressure greater than physiologic saline.

hypertrophy increase in the size of an organ by a process of enlargement of its cells.

hyperventilation abnormally rapid breathing with excessive removal of carbon dioxide, hypocapnia.

hypnosis a state of altered consciousness. The person acts under the influence of a taught suggestion. Can be used as a method for coping with labour.

hypnotherapy treatment based on hypnosis. Labour pains can be controlled in some women by altering their level of consciousness.

hypnotic a drug which induces sleep.

hypo- combining term meaning below normal or under.

hypocalcaemia reduction in the amount of calcium in the circulation.

hypochlorhydria reduction in the amount of hyperchloric acid in the gastric juice.

hypochondrium the right or left upper lateral region of the abdomen, beneath the ribs.

hypochromic reduction in colour or pigment. Description of the iron-deficient erythrocyte as seen in anaemia.

hypodermic 1. subcutaneous. 2. a substance or medicine injected or introduced beneath the skin.

hypofibrinogenaemia a reduction in the plasma level of fibrinogen.

hypogastric relating to the hypogastrium or pubic region.

hypogastric artery a branch from the internal iliac artery which in fetal life carries deoxygenated blood and communicates directly with the umbilical artery.

hypoglycaemia a reduction of glucose in the circulation.

hypognathia having an abnormally small lower jaw.

hypopituitarism clinical condition resulting in reduced secretion from the anterior pituitary gland. It may occur secondary to severe postpartum haemorrhage when there is pituitary necrosis (Sheehan's syndrome), with atrophy of the gonads, thyroid and adrenal glands and secondary infertility.

hypoplasia arrested development of a tissue or organ.

hypospadias a congenital malformation in which the urethra opens on the side surface of the penis or into the vaginal canal.

hypostasis formation of deposits or sedimentation.

hypostatic 1. resulting from hypostasis. 2. a state of being suppressed. In genetics this relates to the genetic characteristic or function that is overshadowed by another gene (of the matched pair), affecting or influencing its functional ability.

hypostatic pneumonia pneumonia developing in the sick patient whose respirations are shallow and who is immobile for long periods.

hypotension abnormally low vessel tension resulting in reduction of blood pressure.

hypothalamus the region of the brain forming the floor of the third ventricle. It controls sympathetic and parasympathetic nervous systems, pituitary activity and various other bodily functions.

hypothermia subnormal body temperature – below 33°C.

hypothermia neonatorum body temperature below 35°C usually as a result of the infant being born in a cool room or inadequately cared for or dried at birth.

hypothesis a conjecture or theory put forward to account for known facts or as a basis for discussion.

hypothyroidism reduction in the functional state of the thyroid gland and insufficiency in production of hormones resulting in cretinism in a child or myxoedema in the adult.

hypotonia reduction in muscle tone.

hypotonic solution a solution that is weaker than physiologic saline and contains less than 0.9 g of sodium chloride per 100 ml.

hypoventilation reduction in respiratory effort.

hypovolaemia marked reduction in the circulating blood volume.

hypovolaemic shock shock or collapsed state resulting from trauma caused by excessive loss of blood or plasma.

hypoxia reduction in oxygen level required for normal physiologic function.

hysterectomy surgical removal of the uterus.

hysterotomy surgical incision into the uterus made for termination of a pregnancy after 12 weeks' but before 28 weeks' gestation.

Ii

iatrogenic a pathological condition caused by treatment given for another condition.

icterus neonatorum jaundice (yellow skin membranes and sclera) of the newborn.

idiopathic primary; of unknown cause.

idiosyncrasy a peculiarity of character or temperament which makes an individual different from others.

Ig symbol for particular gamma globulins, Ig A, D, E, G and M, which offer immunological protection against specific organisms.

ileocaecal valve the valve situated at the junction of the ileum with the caecum that partially prevents reflux.

ileum the terminal section of the small intestine.

ileus intestinal obstruction caused by paralysis of the ileum in which peristalsis is arrested and distension occurs.

iliac pertaining to the ilium or ilial region.

iliac crest the thickened expanded upper border of the hip bone.

iliac fossa the wide shallow depression on the inner surface of the ilium.

iliococcygeal referring to the ilium and coccyx.

iliopectineal referring to the ilium and pubic bone.

ilium the superior widened portion of the hip bone.

immature not yet fully developed.

immature baby a neonate born prematurely, before body systems are developed enough to ensure its survival outside the uterus.

immersion putting into or covering with water. Women may use a bath or birth pool in labour to reduce pain and enhance coping mechanisms by equalizing internal uterine and external pressure.

immobilization removal of capacity of movement. Immobilization due to epidural or general anaesthetic causes the woman to be vulnerable to complications such as deep vein thrombosis.

immune protected against a particular disease.

immune response a reaction involving specific antibody response to an antigen.

immune system the body's natural defence against disease, comprising the biochemical complex of antibodies and T cells, etc., which respond to and protect the body from some infections (*see* Figure 64).

immunity the ability of an organism to mount an antibody response to resist disease.

immunization the active process of developing immunity; the giving of substances in the hope of helping a person develop immunity to one or more diseases.

immunodeficient the failure of the immune system to protect the body from damage by common pathogenic organisms.

immunoglobulin (ABBREVIATION Ig) proteins or gamma globulins having known antibody

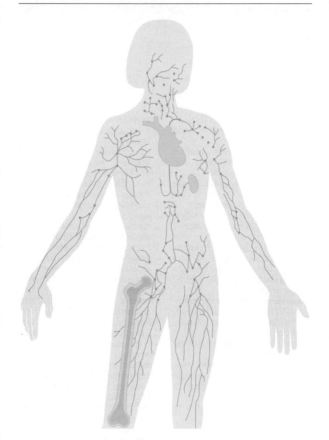

■ **Figure 64** Immune system

activity (IgA, IgD, IgE, IgG, IgM).

immunologic pregnancy test a means of detecting the presence of a pregnancy by measuring the increased concentration of human chorionic gonadotrophin in urine.

immunoprophylaxis a process of hastening immunity by giving live weakened pathogens to an individual or passive immunity through transfer of antibodies made in another body.

impaction being lodged or wedged into a confined space.

impaired glucose tolerance abnormally raised fasting blood glucose levels or failure to return

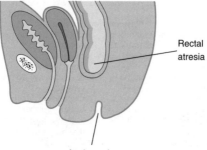

Rectal
atresia

Anal canal

■ **Figure 65** Imperforate anus

to normal parameters within 2 hours of a glucose tolerance test (GTT). May be due to gestational diabetes.

imperforate without the normal opening.

imperforate anus congenital occlusion of the anal opening (*see* Figure 65).

imperforate hymen the absence of a natural opening in the hymen membrane covering the vagina preventing escape of menstrual blood.

impetigo streptococcal or staphylococcal infection of the skin characterized by vesicles which burst exposing erythematous areas. Severe affliction is known as pemphigus neonatorum and is a highly infectious condition.

impetigo herpetiformis a skin condition starting in pregnancy. It resembles a pustular psoriasis with lesions in the genitofemoral area which may spread to other areas.

implant to embed or introduce into the body tissue; something which is embedded or introduced into the body tissue.

implantation 1. the act of implanting, as in the embedding

of the fertilized ovum into the endometrium. 2. the enclosing of drugs such as hormones or radioactive substances in rods, which are then buried under the skin enabling slow release for treatment of certain conditions.

impotent incapable of performing the sexual act.

impregnate to make pregnant.

in utero within the uterus.

in vitro literally, in glass. Used in reference to a process of culture or growth within a test tube.

in vitro fertilization (IVF) fertilization of the ovum outside the female body. Sperm and ovum are removed from their donors, mixed in a glass dish and after fertilization has occurred the conceptus is reintroduced into the uterus for implantation and development to occur.

inborn characteristics that are inherited or congenital.

inborn error of metabolism an inherited genetic characteristic whereby the infant is unable to synthesize foods into simple compounds for ingestion and energy production due to lack of specific enzymes, as in e.g. phenylketonuria and galactosaemia.

inbreeding mating between closely related family members permitting genes and traits to be expressed most strongly in the offspring.

incarcerate enclose, confine or imprison.

incarceration of the retroverted gravid uterus pregnancy conceived with the uterus in the retroverted position which has failed to spontaneously correct, leading to entrapment of the enlarging uterus in the hollow of the sacrum by the sacral promontory.

incest sexual intercourse which is illegal because it is between close members of a family who by law are unable to marry.

incision a cutting into.

incompatibility antagonistic chemical changes resulting when two substances are put together that are not conducive to successful combination.

incompetence inadequacy at the level of normal functional performance.

incompetent cervix ineffective closure of the cervical os secondary to damage of the structure by repeated stretching, as in termination of pregnancy, and resulting in repeated early pregnancy loss.

incomplete abortion describes the situation where some products of conception remain in the uterus after some have been expelled. Surgical removal may be offered to prevent the possibility of infection.

incontinence involuntary and inappropriate passage of waste due to inability to control the anal or urethral sphincter muscles.

incoordinate lacking the harmonious working relationship of various parts.

incubate to artificially heat as a means of bringing about development.

incubation the process of development.

incubation period the time from exposure to an infectious disease to exhibition of symptoms.

incubator 1. a cabinet with controlled temperature used for assisting growth of bacteria or hatching of eggs. 2. a chamber that is closely regulated for temperature, humidity and oxygen in which sick or low birth weight babies are cared for (*see* Figure 66).

independent midwife a midwife who is self-employed and offers continuity of care to women outside of a National Health Service institution. In the UK, most independent midwives primarily work with women wanting home births.

indirect Coombs' test a screening test performed to detect free antibodies in blood. A rhesus negative mother may have this test (or the direct Coombs') done to detect antibodies indicating that the neonate is rhesus positive.

induced abortion intentional termination of pregnancy by drugs or surgical means.

induction the act of bringing about a particular action. Applied to procedures such as abortion, anaesthesia or labour.

induction of labour intentional stimulation of a pregnant uterus to initiate labour using drugs or surgical means.

inertia an ineffective level of activity or sluggishness.

inevitable abortion having reached a stage at which prevention of an abortion is unavoidable.

infant a child up to 12 months of age.

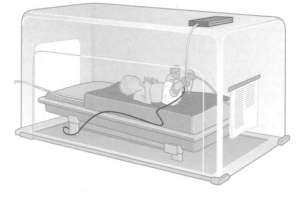

Figure 66 Incubator

infant death death of a child within the first year of life.

infant feeding any method employed for providing nutrition in liquid form to the very young child.

infant mortality rate the number of deaths per year in children under the age of 1 year per 1000 live births.

infanticide the murder of an infant.

infantile 1. pertaining to the period of infancy. 2. having characteristics like those exhibited in infancy.

infantile paralysis poliomyelitis.

infarct ischaemia or necrosis of tissue due to inadequate blood supply.

infarction the development of an infarct.

infected septic abortion termination of pregnancy complicated by invasion of the genital tract with pathogenic organisms. This can be life-threatening; antibiotics and evacuation of the uterus are required.

infection the pathogenic state caused by entry of a micro-organism into a host.

infectious disease a contagious illness caused by an organism invading a host.

inferior below or under.

inferior longitudinal sinus a blood vessel passing around and below the sagittal suture between the parietal bones of the skull.

inferior vena cava the large blood vessel at the lower edge of the falx cerebri.

infertility an involuntary inability to conceive.

infiltrate entry and dispersal of agents into tissue.

inflammation reaction of tissues to injury. Characteristic responses are heat, swelling, redness, pain and loss or reduction of functional ability.

influenza an acute respiratory infection caused by a virus.

informed consent permission for treatment voluntarily obtained from women; the woman must have received a detailed explanation of what is involved, including risks and benefits, in a manner that she is able to understand.

informed refusal refusal of a procedure or treatment which has been offered to a woman, after her consideration of the benefits, risks and alternatives.

infra- a prefix meaning below.

infundibulum (PLURAL infundibula) resembling a funnel; a funnel-shaped passage, for example the distal end of the fallopian tube.

infusion 1. extraction of the soluble properties of a substance by means of soaking in water, but without boiling. 2. slow injection of solution into the body by the intravenous or subcutaneous route.

ingestion 1. the taking in of food or other substances by the oral route. 2. the process by which specialized cells take in or envelop bacteria.

inguinal pertaining to the groin region (inguen).

inguinal canal a small channel running obliquely downwards through the abdominal wall and towards the groin which enables passage of nerves and ligaments. It is also the migratory route taken by the testes in their descent into the scrotal sac.

inguinal hernia descent or herniation of abdominal content into the inguinal canal.

inhalation the process of breathing in a gas or vapour for medicinal or therapeutic purposes, as with Entonox® during labour.

inheritance characteristics genetically acquired from a parent.

inhibin a testicular hormone.

inhibition a restraining of action in an organ or cell.

injection the introduction of fluids into the skin, muscle, blood vessel, spinal cord or any body cavity.

inlet the entrance to a cavity, for example the pelvic inlet or entrance to the true pelvis.

innate present at birth, hereditary, genetically determined.

inner cell mass the compact group of cells that are part of the blastocyst from which the fetus and amniotic membranes develop.

innominate literally, nameless. The *innominate bone* is the collective name given to the bones of the pelvic girdle. It combines the fusion of the ilium, ischium and os pubis (*see* Figure 67).

inoculate to introduce agents derived from a diseased animal or plant into the body of a healthy person for the pur-pose of giving protection against that same disease, e.g. a vaccine.

inquest a legal enquiry for the purpose of determining the cause of sudden, violent or unexplained death.

inquiry based learning (IBL) an approach to education which enables students to determine their own learning needs and seek the information they need. The approach is similar to problem based learning (PBL), with the different term used by some educators and institutions to reflect the fact that midwives mainly work with women who do not have problems.

insemination 1. the planting of seed. 2. the introduction of seminal fluid into the female genital tract for the purpose of achieving conception.

insertion the anchorage point of a muscle or the attachment of an organ to its support.

insidious gradual development or progression of a condition or disease so as to be almost imperceptible.

insomnia inability to sleep.

inspection to look at or examine visually, e.g. before abdominal palpation.

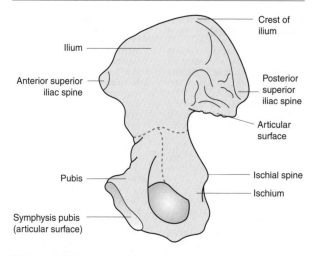

Crest of
ilium

Ilium

Anterior superior
iliac spine

Posterior
superior
iliac spine

Articular
surface

Pubis

Ischial spine

Ischium

Symphysis pubis
(articular surface)

■ **Figure 67** Innominate bone

inspiration inhalation, drawing in of breath.

instillation introduction of a liquid into a cavity or canal drop by drop.

instrument a tool with a specific purpose.

instrumental delivery the use of an instrument or tool to aid birth, e.g. ventouse, forceps.

insufficiency the inability to perform at the optimal level of function.

insufflation the introduction of gas, powder or vapour into a body cavity by blowing or positive pressure.

insulin 1. the hypoglycaemic hormone secreted by the beta cells of the islets of Langerhans in the pancreas which regulates carbohydrate and fat metabolism. 2. a synthetic drug which replaces endogenous insulin.

intelligence quotient (IQ) a numerical rating used to designate a person's cognitive skill (understanding) as compared to the average for age and social situation.

intensive care unit a designated area where the critically ill patient can be observed and monitored constantly and receive additional supportive care and therapy from specially qualified persons.

intention to practise documentation completed by each midwife at the commencement of work and annually, ensuring the availability of a local and up-to-date list of midwives competent to practise.

inter- prefix denoting between.

intercellular between cells.

intercostal between the ribs.

intercourse communication or interaction. *Sexual intercourse* (coitus) is penetration of the vagina by the penis and ejaculation.

interface a surface that forms a boundary between two opposing units.

interferon a protein formed by cells in response to a virus which prevents future viral replication and can induce resistance to a range of other viruses.

interleukin-8 a low molecular weight protein involved in cell-to-cell communication, coordination of antibodies, T cell immune interactions and the inflammatory process; it may have some effect on the commencement of labour.

intermenstrual referring to the time between menstrual periods.

intermittent occurring at intervals or periodically.

intermittent positive pressure ventilation (IPPV) mechanical ventilation of the lungs, often employed in babies with severe respiratory distress syndrome.

internal os the innermost opening or mouth at the junction of the uterine cavity with the cervix.

internal podalic version a procedure where the operator's hand is introduced into the uterus to apply pressure to convert an undeliverable malpresentation (e.g. shoulder presentation) to one which may be more safely delivered vaginally (breech) by bringing the feet down so that they are the presenting part. (*See* internal version.)

internal rotation of the fetus in the second stage of labour, when the cervix is fully dilated, this is part of the mechanism performed by the fetus as it adapts to the changing shape and diameters of the birth canal.

internal version manipulation of the fetus in utero to alter the lie from oblique to longitudinal when the breech presents or to correct a brow presentation. One hand is inserted into the uterus while the other works externally over the abdomen (*see* Figure 68).

interrupted not continuous. An *interrupted suture* is a type of wound closure in which each stitch is tied and cut before the next one is applied.

intersex an individual of indeterminable gender, being either a pseudo- or true hermaphrodite.

interspinous situated between or connecting bony protrusions.

interstitial relating to the space between organs filled by fine connective tissue.

interstitial fibroid a fibroid which develops and is located within the intercellular connective tissue layers of the uterus.

interstitial mastitis inflammation of the connective tissue between the ducts of the breast.

interstitial tubal pregnancy a pregnancy which has implanted in the narrowest part of the fallopian tube.

intervillous situated between villi.

intestinal flora the naturally occurring non-pathogenic micro-organisms found in the large intestine and responsible for the manufacture of vitamin K and other useful substances.

intestinal obstruction spasmodic and inflammatory constriction of the gut causing blockage and preventing material passing through. It causes pain, distension, tenderness and constitutes a medical emergency often requiring emergency surgery.

intestine the part of the digestive tract extending from the stomach to the anus.

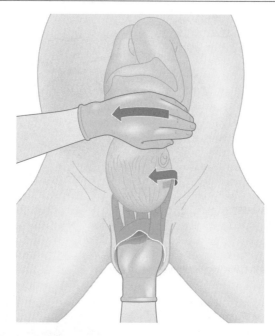

■ **Figure 68** Internal version

intra- prefix denoting within or inward.

intra-abdominal pressure pressure within the abdomen from accumulation of gases, faecal material, infection or pregnancy.

intracerebral haemorrhage bleeding inside the brain (*see* Figure 69).

intracranial inside the head.

intracranial haemorrhage bleeding within the skull; can occur in the neonate following an instrumental or vaginal breech delivery.

intracranial pressure a rise from the normal pressure level caused by an accumulation of blood or fluid under the skull, recognized by falling pulse rate and rising blood pressure, increased restlessness and a decrease in the level of consciousness.

intradermal into or within the skin. An *intradermal injection* is one given between the epidermis and the dermis (*see* Figure 70).

intramenstrual pain uterine pain between menstrual periods; there may be an association with ovulation.

intramuscular into or within a muscle. An *intramuscular injection* is one given into a muscle (*see* Figure 71).

intrapartum occurring during parturition or childbirth.

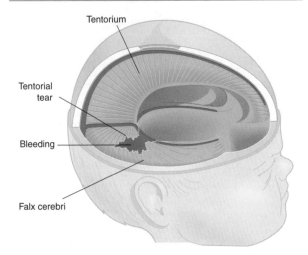

Figure 69 Intracerebral haemorrhage

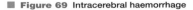

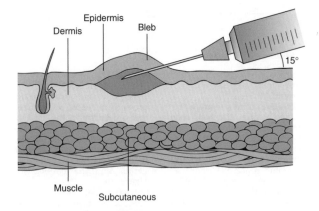

Figure 70 Intradermal injection technique

intrapartum haemorrhage bleeding from the genital tract during labour; may be associated with placenta praevia or abruptio placentae.

intrauterine within the uterus.
intrauterine contraceptive device (IUCD) mechanical device inserted within the uterine cavity which prevents

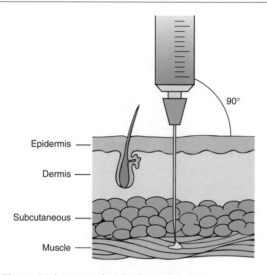

Epidermis ——

Dermis ——

Subcutaneous ——

Muscle ——

▓ Figure 71 Intramuscular injection technique

implantation or development of the fertilized embryo (*see* Figure 72).

intrauterine death (IUD) death of the fetus while in the uterus.

intrauterine growth restriction (IUGR) previously known as *intrauterine growth retardation* failure of the fetus to develop in accordance with recognized growth curves with regard to increasing weight, size and bone length.

intravascular within the blood vessels.

intravascular coagulation clotting of blood within the blood vessels. They may then cause other vessels to become obstructed, e.g. in the kidney, and damage in that organ may be permanent. The clotting factors will become unbalanced and haemorrhage is possible.

intravenous (IV; i.v.) within or into a vein.

intravenous infusion (IVI) introduction of a fluid into the body, e.g. for hydration, to increase circulating volume before introduction of a potentially hypotensive drug, as a circulatory expander, or for nutritional purposes.

intravenous injection a drug or medicine introduced directly into the circulatory system so that the time for it to take effect is short.

intraventricular haemorrhage bleeding into the ventricles deep within the brain. It can happen to preterm infants or those experiencing a traumatic delivery. Often results in permanent physical or mental disability.

intrinsic situated or produced within a part, relating to inherent factor within itself.

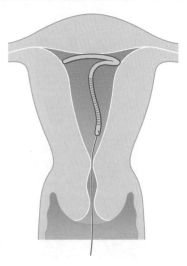

Figure 72 Intrauterine contraceptive device (IUCD)

intrinsic factor a substance produced by the stomach which, when combined with properties of food (vitamin B$_{12}$, the extrinsic factor) is essential to prevent pernicious anaemia.

introitus an entrance; the term is often used to refer to the opening of the vagina.

intubation the introduction of a tube into a hollow organ. *Endotracheal intubation* is used to achieve mechanical ventilation in cases of neonatal asphyxia or in association with induction of anaesthesia.

intussusception the prolapse of the bowel either into itself or through the rectum.

invasion the process whereby a disease or pathogen enters, infects and damages the body.

inverse, inverted located in the opposite position from that which it is normally expected; turned inwards or upside down.

inversion turning inside out. *Uterine inversion* is a rare but serious complication of the third stage of labour (*see* Figure 73); it causes profound shock.

inverted *see* inverse.

involuntary acting independently of will or conscious control.

involution a process of regression which some organs undergo, having fulfilled their intended function.

involution of the uterus return of the uterus to its non-pregnant condition (*see* Figure 74).

ion an atom or group of atoms which by application of an energy source can gain or lose electrons and be rendered capable of conducting electricity.

iron an organic metal used in the form of salts in medicines for the treatment of anaemia. It is essential in the manufacture of haemoglobin.

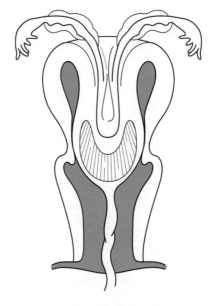

■ **Figure 73** Inversion of the uterus

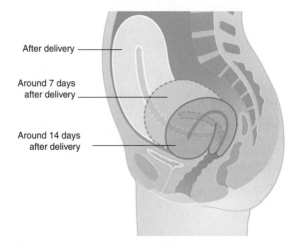

After delivery

Around 7 days
after delivery

Around 14 days
after delivery

■ **Figure 74** Involution of the uterus

ischaemia diminution of blood supply to an area of the body.

ischaemic necrosis tissue death occurring secondary to lack of an adequate blood supply.

ischial relating to the ischium.

ischial spine the bony prominence on the ischium which protrudes into the pelvic cavity.

ischial tuberosity the rounded lower border of the ischium on which the body rests when sitting.

ischiocavernosus muscle muscle from the ischium to the clitoris or penis.

ischiococcygeus muscle muscle from the ischium to the coccyx.

ischium the inferior and posterior dense portion of the innominate bone upon which the body rests when in a sitting position.

islets of Langerhans the endocrine structures of the pancreas which produce insulin. Insulin controls carbohydrate metabolism. In the disease diabetes mellitus the islets fail.

isoimmunization sensitization of a species with antigens from the same species. This can occur in mismatched blood transfusion or where a woman is rhesus negative and the fetus rhesus positive. Fetal blood cells can pass into the maternal circulation which may cause her to produce antibodies against the foreign cells. The antibodies she produces can cross the placenta, entering the fetal circulation and causing haemolysis.

isolation separation of an infective individual from the remainder of the community to contain and prevent the spread of a communicable disease to others.

isotonic relating to uniformity of strength.

isotonic solution solution containing the same osmotic pressure as the tissue with which it is compared and capable of promoting or maintaining its normal state or function. Physiologic normal saline is isotonic with plasma.

isthmus the constricted part or neck of an organ.

Jj

Jacquemier's sign blue discoloration of the vaginal lining seen in early pregnancy and taken as one of the presumed diagnostic signs.

jaundice yellow discoloration of the skin, mucous membranes and sclera due to hyperbilirubinaemia.

joint the point at which two or more bones meet.

joint instability the effects of the hormones progesterone and relaxin on the joints in pregnancy causing them to soften and have an increased range of movement, e.g. the sacroiliac joint and the symphysis pubis.

joule (J) the international unit of energy measurement in food.

jugular relating to the neck or region above the clavicle.

justice ethical principle which recognizes fairness and equality of treatment for all.

justo minor abnormally small in all dimensions. A term applied to the perfectly formed but small gynaecoid pelvis.

juvenile young adult, youth.

juxta- prefix denoting nearness or proximity to, as in *juxtaposition*.

Kk

K symbol for potassium.

Kahn test blood test for syphilis.

kallikrein a proteolytic enzyme present in several body fluids that releases kallidin.

kangaroo care a method of caring for the neonate derived from the Australian marsupial in which the immature offspring is carried and suckled in a pouch on the mother's abdomen. It has been found to be physiologically beneficial.

Kaposi's sarcoma multiple, idiopathic haemorrhagic sarcoma lesions, often seen as a feature of AIDS.

karyo- combining form denoting nucleus.

karyogenesis formation and development of cell nuclei.

karyotype the total characteristics including numbers, size and form of chromosomes and their grouping in a cell nucleus.

Kell blood group a family of antigens found in erythrocytes in a small percentage of the population [K, k, Kp, Kp and Ku].

keloid fibrous tissue hyperplasia formed at the site of a scar.

keratin an albuminous substance forming the base of all horny tissues (hair, nails, feathers, etc.).

kernicterus bilirubin hyperpigmentation of the basal ganglia of the brain with destruction of nerve cells, seen as a complication of severe neonatal jaundice caused by rhesus isoimmunization.

Kernig's sign pain and spasm of the hamstring muscles resulting in an inability of a supine patient to straighten the leg when it is flexed at the knee and hip – a sign of meningitis.

ketoacidosis accumulation of ketone bodies and acetic acid in the blood. This can occur when the body is starved of a ready supply of energy and breaks down body stores of fats leading to the production of toxic metabolites.

ketone body acetone formed by the metabolism of fats.

ketonuria the presence of ketone bodies in the urine.

ketosis condition in which excessive amounts of ketones are present in the body.

ketotic presence of ketones in the body as indicated by acidic expired air and ketonuria.

kick chart a graphical record made by a pregnant woman indicating the number of fetal movements counted during a designated time period; may be used as an assessment of fetal well-being.

Kielland's forceps an obstetric forceps, characterized by reduced curvature of the blades and interlocking handles. Used for mid-cavity application and rotation of the fetal head.

killed vaccine an injection of dead micro-organisms to which the body responds by producing antibodies.

kinase an enzyme that catalyses transfer of phosphate from adenosine triphosphate to an acceptor.

kinin any of a group of polypeptides capable of initiating capillary wall activity. Bradykinin (causes relaxation of capillary walls) is mainly hypotensive while angiotensin (causes constriction of capillary walls) is hypertensive.

Kleihauer test a blood test performed on the rhesus negative mother to detect the presence of fetal cells in the maternal circulation. Where detected and the fetus is identified as rhesus positive, anti-D immunoglobulin is offered to the mother in an attempt to prevent isoimmunization.

Klinefelter's syndrome a clinical syndrome in males characterized by having an additional sex chromosome (XXY instead of XY). The testes fail to mature at puberty and there may be female characteristics such as the development of breasts.

Klumpke's paralysis paralysis of the forearm and hand caused by damage to the lower brachial nerve plexus. A birth injury often associated with excessive traction on the neck to deliver the anterior shoulder.

knee–chest position a position assumed by the woman in which she rests on forearms and knees with hips elevated. Most often adopted when there is a cord presentation or prolapse, or where there is a need to encourage the presenting part out of the pelvis, e.g. to help the baby rotate and re-enter in a more favourable position.

knee presentation a variation of breech presentation in which one or both knees of the fetus precede the buttocks.

'know your midwife' scheme the model of care offered by a team of midwives in Tooting, London, as a pilot study to discover the advantages and disadvantages of the scheme and to be a model for future teams.

Kocher's forceps surgical forceps with serrated jaws and sharp interlocking teeth at the lips. Occasionally used to artificially rupture the fetal membranes.

Koplik's spots white spots inside the mouth – the first sign of measles infection.

Korotkoff method a means of determining the diastolic blood pressure reading. There are four Korotkoff sounds distinguishable as the diastolic sound diminishes. Midwives should note which sound they record as it makes a difference to the diagnosis of pregnancy-induced hypertension (PIH).

Krukenberg's tumour bilateral metastatic carcinoma of the ovaries, usually secondary to gastric carcinoma.

kyphosis convex, deformed curvature of the spine resulting in a hump on the back.

LI

La Leche League a voluntary organization that promotes and provides education and support for mothers wishing to breastfeed.

labia (SINGULAR labium) the two fleshy folds of skin on either side of the opening to the vagina. Labia majora are the outer fleshy folds; labia minora are the inner skin folds.

labial referring to the labia.

labile unstable, not fixed, subject to variations. Will change to different values at different times.

labour (SYNONYMS parturition, childbirth) the process of giving birth. Artificially divided into three stages. The first stage of labour refers to the dilation of the cervical os to 10 cm. The second stage is from the full dilation of the cervical os to the complete birth of the baby. The third stage of labour refers to the expulsion of the placenta and membranes.

labour coach a person who assists a woman in labour and delivery by encouraging her to use previously taught techniques such as breathing patterns, concentration, positions, and the employment of massage.

laboured breathing respiration which is difficult, noisy and uses all ancillary respiratory muscles. Present in preterm neonates with respiratory distress syndrome.

laceration a tear or injury.

lacrimal referring to the tears. The *lacrimal ducts* (*see* Figure 75)

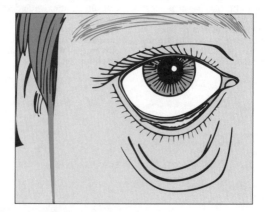

■ **Figure 75** Lacrimal duct

are part of the drainage system that carries tears from the *lacrimal glands*, the tear-secreting glands, to the nose.

lactalbumin the most important protein in human breast milk.

lactase an enzyme produced by the small intestine which splits lactose into monosaccharides glucose and galactose.

lactation the secretion of milk by the breasts.

lacteals the lymphatic vessels surrounding the intestines which absorb split fats.

lactic acid an acid which is formed when there is a reduction in the amount of oxygen available for use in the body (hypoxic episodes). It causes the blood to become more acid (acidaemia). It is also found in the vagina and is produced by the action of bacilli on lactose. The acid climate created protects against some pathogenic organisms.

lactiferous duct one of the many tiny channels which carry breast milk from the mammary lobes which open on to the nipple.

Lactobacillus acidophilus (SYNONYM Döderlein's bacillus) bacteria which grow in the vagina and convert glycogen to lactic acid which is said to prevent the growth of other organisms. It is also found in the stools of breastfed babies and has the same function.

lactoferrin the iron-binding protein found in human milk. It protects the infant from infection caused by the *Escherichia coli* bacterium.

lactogen a substance which enables lactation. *Human placental lactogen* is a hormone secreted by the placenta which promotes growth and inhibits insulin's activity during pregnancy.

lactoglobulin a protein found in milk.

lactose a sugar found in milk. *Lactose intolerance* occurs when there is not enough lactase to split the sugar so it can be absorbed for use in the body. The condition causes diarrhoea and failure to thrive and is treated by giving lactose-free milk.

lactulose a mild medicine given by mouth to treat constipation; it may take up to 48 hours to be effective.

laked describes blood that has haemolysed (erythrocytes which have split into their iron and protein components) due to severe infection, poisoning or burns.

Lamaze method preparation for childbirth developed by a French obstetrician based on a psychoprophylactic technique for changing the brain's perception of pain.

Lamba sign seen by ultrasound as a thickened area of placental tissue at the site of insertion of the separating membranes suggesting a dichorionic placentation and non-identical twins.

lambda the posterior fontanelle which may be felt at the back of the fetal skull.

lambdoidal suture the crease felt at the side of the fetal skull running between the occipital bone and the parietal bone.

lamellar exfoliation of the newborn a congenital abnormality in which the infant is born with a scaly membrane over the skin. It peels off within 48 hours of birth.

lancet a short, pointed blade used to obtain a drop of blood for a capillary sample.

Langerhans islets *see* islets of Langerhans.

Langhans' cell layer the inside layer of the trophoblast.

lanolin the fat on (mainly) sheep's wool which is the basis for ointments.

lanugo the fine hair which covers the fetus in utero and is shed into the liquor just before term.

laparoscopic sterilization a surgical procedure in which clips are applied to the fallopian tubes through a small incision in the abdomen. The sperm's passage towards the ovum is blocked, thereby preventing pregnancy.

laparotomy an opening made into a body cavity to examine the contents.

Largactil® (chlorpromazine) a drug used as a sedative.

large for gestational age a fetus whose growth is greater than the 90th percentile. May be caused by genetic factors, maternal diabetes or Beckwith's syndrome.

laryngoscope an instrument used to inspect the larynx and vocal cords. It aids insertion of an endotracheal tube which gives access to the lungs.

larynx the voice box, part of the air passages situated between the trachea and the base of the tongue.

Lasix® (furosemide (frusemide)) a drug which decreases circulating volume in the blood by increasing urinary output.

last menstrual period (LMP) the date of the first day of the last normal menses. It is used to estimate the possible date of birth of a baby using Nägele's rule.

latent hidden.

latent activity changes which are happening but are not apparent, e.g. in the very early stages of labour.

latent period, latent phase seemingly inactive phase of early labour when contractions are less efficient and cervical dilation is slow.

lateral referring to the side.

latex the sap of certain plants containing resins, proteins and other substances used to make rubber. It can cause allergic reactions in some individuals.

lavender oil an oil made from lavender flowers which has therapeutic properties. May be used to aid perineal healing and reduce discomfort in labour.

laxative a mild medicine which promotes bowel evacuation by increasing the bulk of the faeces, softening the stool or lubricating the intestinal walls.

lead professional the qualified person who takes prime responsibility for the care of a pregnant and postpartum woman. This person may be a midwife, GP or obstetrician, according to the woman's wishes. Other professionals may be involved.

learning improving the performance of psychomotor skill, attitudes or cognitive skills.

Leboyer method a very calm, quiet, darkened, warm environment is created around the birth of the baby. Leboyer, a French obstetrician, considered that this minimized the trauma of birth for both parents and child thereby creating greater satisfaction with the process.

lecithin a molecule made of a protein and a fat which is found in the alveoli of the lungs. It acts as a surfactant, which helps to keep the lungs open. The amount of this substance can be measured in amniotic fluid as an indicator of fetal maturity and likelihood of respiratory distress syndrome developing after delivery.

lecturer a person who has spent time gaining specialist knowledge in her sphere of interest and who will talk to others from a position of expertise.

Lee–Frankenhauser plexus a network of nerves serving the

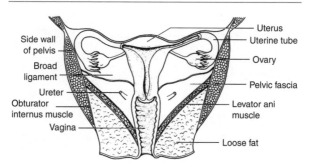

■ **Figure 76** Levator ani

cervix and pelvic cavity region of the body.

Leeds test (SYNONYM triple test) a screening test like Bart's test which identifies women at high risk of carrying a fetus with Down's syndrome. It measures alphafetoprotein, unconjugated oestriol, human chorionic gonadotrophin, and neutrophil alkaline phosphatase. It indicates whether a diagnostic test such as amniocentesis may be of value to an individual woman.

lesion 1. an injury or wound to a part of the body. 2. any structural abnormality or pathologic change in tissues.

'let-down' reflex the release of breast milk to the nipple when the lactiferous ducts contract. It is initiated by the baby sucking or crying.

leucocyte *see* leukocyte.

leucorrhoea a white mucoid, inoffensive vaginal discharge. The amount is increased in pregnancy, at ovulation and during sexual arousal.

leukocyte (leucocyte) a white blood corpuscle (cell).

levallorphan (levorphanol) a drug which works in oppos-

ition to analgesic narcotic drugs such as pethidine.

levator a strong muscle which raises and supports.

levator ani three muscles which stretch across the pelvic floor (*see* Figure 76). They are the main support of the abdominal and pelvic organs.

liability something one is obligated to do, or for which one must be accountable; an obligation under law, a responsibility.

libido desire for sexual intercourse.

lidocaine hydrochloride (lignocaine hydrochloride) a drug which causes analgesia and nerve block to the tissues into which it is injected. Up to 10 ml of a 1% solution may be used by a midwife when performing an episiotomy or a perineal repair.

lie the relationship of the long axis of the fetus (spine) to the long axis (spine) of the mother. When they are parallel the lie is said to be longitudinal; when the fetal spine is across the mother's spine, the lie is transverse; and when the fetus is diagonal to the mother's spine

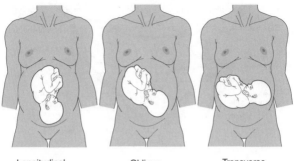

| Longitudinal | Oblique | Transverse |

■ **Figure 77** Lie – longitudinal, oblique, transverse

the lie is oblique (*see* Figure 77).

ligament a tough band of fibrous tissue connecting bones together or supporting organs.

ligature a thread – catgut, Vicryl, or nylon – used for tying off blood vessels so they do not bleed.

light for dates *see* small for gestational age.

lightening the sensation experienced by women in late pregnancy when the fetus settles lower in the pelvis leaving more space in the upper abdomen.

linea alba the middle line of the abdomen representing the fusion of three strong sheets of fibrous tissue which cover the front of the abdomen.

linea nigra the pigmented line which appears during pregnancy, developing from the symphysis pubis upwards. The line fades slowly after pregnancy.

Lippes Loop an intrauterine contraceptive device.

liquor (liquor amnii) the fluid which surrounds the fetus and fills out the uterine cavity. It is thought to be secreted by the fetal membranes lining the uterus. It is 99% water, with some proteins, fats and carbohydrates, fetal urine, lanugo, vernix and dead fetal cells. It allows growth and movement, acts as a shock absorber and equalizes pressure on the fetus and placenta. There is approximately 1 litre at 37 weeks for an average sized fetus but this decreases towards term.

listeria a gram-negative bacterium which causes upper respiratory infection, septicaemia and encephalitic disease.

lithotomy position the woman lies on her back with her legs flexed, abducted and supported around two lithotomy poles in stirrups. The woman's legs must be lifted together by one person on each side of the bed because the hip joints are very soft due to the hormones in pregnancy and damage can easily occur.

litmus paper thin strips of blotting paper impregnated with the litmus pigment. It is used to find out if fluids are acid or alkaline. Blue litmus is turned red by acids and red litmus is turned blue by alkalis.

live birth an infant of more than 24 weeks' gestation who responds to stimulation at birth and shows all the signs of life.

liver the vital organ situated on the right side of the abdomen slightly under and protected by the ribs. It stores carbohydrates, iron and vitamins; destroys toxins, drugs, alcohol and poisons; makes bile, plasma proteins, antibodies, clotting factors (prothrombin and fibrinogen) and heat.

lobe a section or small part of an organ separated from other parts by fibrous tissue or fissures.

lobule a small lobe or smaller section or segment of a lobe.

local anaesthesia a drug injected into tissue to reduce sensation in the area, e.g. as used before repair of the perineum.

local anaesthetic a drug given to prevent the transmission of impulses through nerves and stop sensation of pain registering in the brain, e.g. epidural anaesthetic.

local authority the local government for a geographical area with regulatory and prosecuting powers.

local supervising authority (LSA) a group of professionals usually within the regional health authority who are responsible for midwifery practice within its area. The LSA appoints a *supervisor of midwives* who monitors the quality of practice, advises in difficult circumstances, and recommends training and direction for developing the midwives she supervises. The supervisor maintains a list of practising midwives, both independent and employed, within her area and may suspend midwives whose practice is deemed unsafe.

lochia the vaginal loss after birth which is made up of blood, dead cells, liquor, vernix, meconium and other debris from the uterus. It changes over the first few days from *lochia rubra*, which is largely fresh blood, to *lochia serosa*, which is pink and contains more white than red blood cells, to *lochia alba*, which is whitish and mainly mucoid. These changes can take up to 3 or 4 weeks. Normal lochia changes progressively and does not smell offensive.

locked twins a rare condition where each twin is preventing the other from being born. Labour will be obstructed (*see* Figure 78).

longitudinal a measurement referring to the longest aspect of a body or organ.

longitudinal lie the long axis of the fetus (spine) is parallel to the long axis of the mother (spine). Presentation can be breech or cephalic.

lordosis a condition where the spine is curved more than the moderate degree seen in pregnancy. Normally the spine curves backwards as the body attempts to accommodate the extra abdominal weight and keep the centre of gravity over the feet. A degree of backache will be experienced.

Lovsett's manoeuvre a technique to delivery of the shoulders when the fetus is presenting by the breech and the arms are above the head. The fetus is rotated half a circle so that the posterior arm is twisted across the face and the elbow can be reached and delivered. The fetus is then rotated half a circle in the reverse direction so that the other arm can be delivered similarly (*see* Figure 79).

low birth weight a baby weighing less than 2.5 kg either because it is preterm or

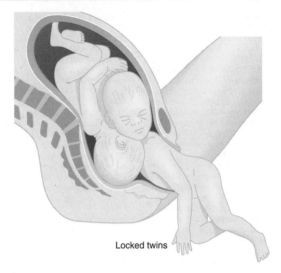

Locked twins

■ **Figure 78** Locked twins

because it is small for gestational age.

lower segment caesarean section (LSCS) an operation during which the lower segment of the uterus is opened surgically from an abdominal wound in order to deliver the baby.

lower uterine segment the part of the uterus lying just above the cervix which will become relaxed, thin and incorporate the cervix during labour.

lubricant a cream or jelly applied to hands, gloves or instruments in order to make them slippery and easier to insert.

lumbar referring to the lower part of the spine.

lumbar puncture a diagnostic or treatment procedure during which a needle is introduced into the subarachnoid space and cerebrospinal fluid withdrawn

or medication introduced (*see* Figure 80). This sometimes occurs accidentally during siting of an epidural and is usually accompanied by severe headaches and neck stiffness. In this case a blood patch may be performed and pushing during the second stage of labour is contraindicated as it would raise the pressure within the spine and cause leakage of cerebrospinal fluid.

luteal referring to the corpus luteum on the outside of the ovary in the second half of the menstrual cycle.

lutein the yellow colour in the corpus luteum.

luteinizing hormone a hormone secreted from the anterior part of the pituitary gland which with follicle stimulating hormone causes ovulation and the formation of the corpus luteum in the

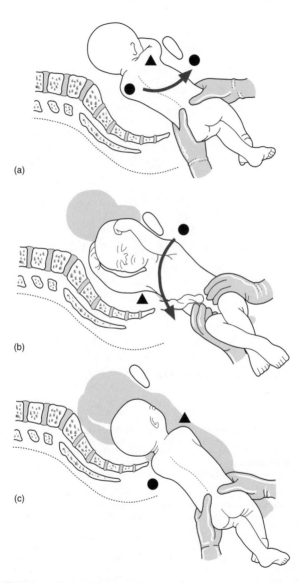

(a)

(b)

(c)

■ **Figure 79** Lovsett's manoeuvre

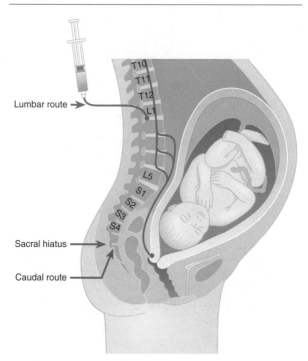

Figure 80 Lumbar puncture

female. In the male it promotes development of the interstitial cells and secretion of testosterone.

lying-in older, colloquial term for the specific period of time just before, during and after childbirth when a woman needs care and rest.

lymph exudate that surrounds the cells which drains into the *lymphatic system* (*see* Figure 81) and then into the blood.

lymphatics the vessels which carry lymph.

lymphocyte white blood cells made in the bone marrow and thymus whose function is to fight infection.

lysis the gradual fall of a fever or breakdown of red blood cells.

lysozyme an antibacterial substance found in tissues, and secreted in tears and breast milk.

lytic cocktail a collection of drugs previously used to manage severe pre-eclampsia. Contains chlorpromazine, promethazine and pethidine.

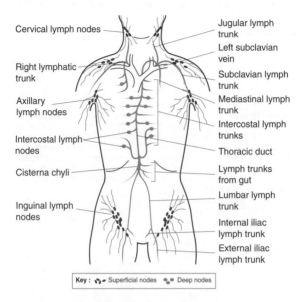

Cervical lymph nodes

Right lymphatic trunk

Axillary lymph nodes

Intercostal lymph nodes

Cisterna chyli

Inguinal lymph nodes

Jugular lymph trunk

Left subclavian vein

Subclavian lymph trunk

Mediastinal lymph trunk

Intercostal lymph trunks

Thoracic duct

Lymph trunks from gut

Lumbar lymph trunk

Internal iliac lymph trunk

External iliac lymph trunk

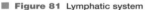

Key : ⬤ Superficial nodes ⬤ Deep nodes

■ **Figure 81 Lymphatic system**

Mm

maceration the process of softening a solid mass by soaking it. A *macerated fetus* is a dead fetus which has soaked in liquor so that it has become soft. Its skin is blue and peels, and it may disintegrate (*see* Figure 82). This indicates that the fetus died before labour. Enzymes released from the tissue may cause a serious complication to the mother called disseminated intravascular coagulation.

Mackenrodt's ligament the transverse or cardinal ligament that supports the uterus at the cervical level within the pelvic cavity.

macrencephaly a large brain, which is usually a congenital condition.

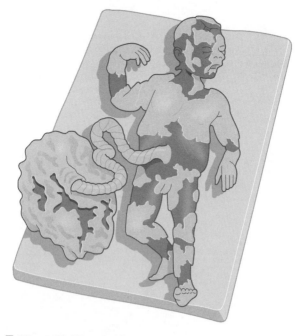

■ **Figure 82** Macerated fetus

macro- combining form meaning large.

macrocephaly a large head and brain in comparison to the rest of the body. Mental and physical retardation are usually present.

macrocyte an abnormally large red blood cell. Macrocytic erythrocytes are found in the blood in megaloblastic anaemia of pregnancy due to lack of folic acid in the diet during their manufacture.

macrogenitosomia enlargement of the external genitalia in boys and pseudohermaphroditism in girls. It is congenital in origin.

macroglossia enlargement of the tongue. A congenital condition, usually seen in Down's syndrome.

macrognathia enlargement of the jaw.

macroscopic visible with the naked eye.

macular rash many small flat red spots on the skin.

magnesium an element essential for life.

magnesium sulphate a salt of magnesium prescribed intravenously to prevent seizures, especially in pre-eclampsia, and by mouth to treat constipation and heartburn (*magnesium trisilicate*). The latter may be given before general anaesthetic to reduce the acidity of the gastric contents and thereby prevent Mendelson's syndrome.

magnetic resonance imaging (MRI) the use of radio frequency radiation as a means of obtaining images of the internal parts of the body.

mal- combining form meaning bad, wrong or ill; a disorder. *Grand mal* is a generalized fit or convulsion, *petit mal* a momentary loss of consciousness without convulsion.

malabsorption inability to absorb nutrients from the intestines. The nutrients will be passed out in the stools (*malabsorption syndrome*).

malaise a feeling of general discomfort, loss of energy or illness.

malaria a tropical infection transmitted through the skin by a mosquito bite. The insect injects a protozoal parasite which develops in the erythrocyte causing anaemia, febrile illness and splenomegaly.

male refers to the sex that produces sperm cells and fertilizes the female ovum (egg) in the process of reproduction.

malformation an anatomical abnormality, either acquired or congenital.

malignant a term applied to a condition which will become progressively degenerative and result in death.

malnutrition a disorder of the diet, either incorrect foods or not enough food.

malposition in the wrong place. Refers to a position of the fetus in the uterus which will not aid normal progress in labour (*see* Figure 83).

malpractice inadequate skills, care or conduct from a professionally qualified person. It can result in injury, suffering or death. Used in law to denote negligence (that which a reasonable person would not do).

malpresentation when the fetal head is not over the cervix; the breech, brow, shoulder or face may be found instead (*see* Figure 84).

maltase an enzyme which splits maltose into glucose. Found in the pancreatic and intestinal juices.

maltose a sugar formed when starch is decomposed by the action of amylase.

mammary referring to the breasts.

mammillary referring to the nipples.

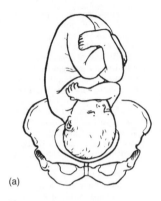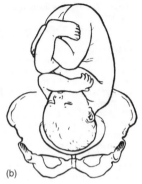

(a)   (b)

■ **Figure 83** Malposition

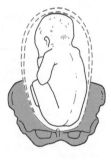

Breech   Shoulder

■ **Figure 84** Malpresentation

mammography X-ray examination of the breasts to look for cancers and other disorders. A contrast medium may be used.

Manchester operation amputation of the cervix with anterior and posterior narrowing of the vagina.

mandelic acid a drug used as an antiseptic in the treatment of urinary tract infections including cystitis, nephritis and pyelitis.

mandible the lower jaw bone.

mania a severe mental disorder which may, rarely, follow childbirth. Associated with rapid, extreme mood swings and possible violence.

manic-depressive psychosis a mental illness characterized by alternating attacks of mania and depression.

manipulation using the hands in a skilled manner to change a position (e.g. the fetus in the uterus or bones in the spine).

manoeuvre a procedure carried out with the hands (e.g. *Lovsett's manoeuvre*).

manometer an instrument used to measure pressure or tension (e.g. of blood in the arteries).

Mantoux test a test to detect immunity to tuberculosis (TB). A small amount of old tuberculin is injected under the skin. A reaction indicates immunity.

manual with the hands.

manual removal of the placenta the removal of the placenta from the uterus by inserting a hand into the uterus and separating the placenta from the uterine wall; this may

be done by a midwife in an emergency (*see* Figure 85).

manual rotation turning of the baby's head from a transverse position by internally applied pressure to dislodge its fixture on the ischial spines and rotating it to a more favourable position, i.e. occipitoanterior or occipitoposterior.

maple syrup urine disease an inherited metabolic disorder. An enzyme necessary for the breakdown of the amino acids valine, leucine and isoleucine is absent. It is recognized in infancy by the odour of the urine, mental and physical handicap and hyperreflexia.

marasmus severe malnutrition and weight loss in babies and infants associated with protein and calorie deficiency.

Marcain® (bupivacaine) a local analgesic put into the epidural

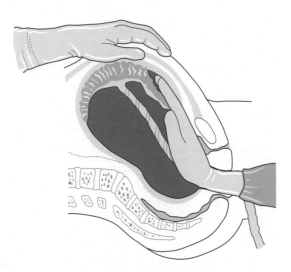

■ **Figure 85** Manual removal of the placenta

space. It causes loss of sensation from the level of the epidural downwards and may cause the blood pressure to fall.

Marevan® (warfarin) tablets given to prevent blood clotting. This anticoagulant drug is given to women with a history of thrombosis.

Marfan's syndrome a hereditary condition recognized by elongation of the bones, often in association with abnormalities of the eyes and cardiovascular system.

marginal placenta praevia a placenta which is low-lying, its edges located on the margin of the lower segment of the uterus, possibly reaching the internal cervical os.

marijuana prepared from the hemp plant *Cannabis sativa*. Hashish is made from the flowers of the same plant. Usually smoked but can be ingested. It gives a feeling of euphoria and may relieve pain. Its possession is illegal.

marrow the fatty, sponge-like material in the cavity of bones. It is responsible for the manufacture of all types of blood cells.

masculine having the characteristics and features of a male.

massage stroking or kneading of the body to aid relaxation, stimulate circulation and excretion, and lower blood pressure. In labour some women like to be stroked over the abdomen or kneaded over the lower spine. *Cardiac massage* is carried out when the heart stops, for the purpose of resuscitation; externally the heart is compressed between the ribs and the spine, or it can be done internally by hand following opening of the chest wall.

mastalgia pain in the breast, for which there are a number of different causes.

mastectomy the excision of the breast, usually done to remove a malignant tumour.

mastitis inflammation of the breasts. Organisms may enter through cracked nipples and a wedge shaped area becomes red, tender and hot. Rapid treatment is required to prevent the formation of an abscess. Breast-feeding is not contraindicated and may aid recovery.

masturbation pleasurable stimulation of the genitals by oneself or with a partner (*mutual masturbation*), often to the point of orgasm.

MAT B1 maternity certificate signed by the midwife or doctor indicating the likely date of delivery. Employers require this certificate in order to award maternity pay.

materia medica the study of drugs – sources, preparations, uses and effects. *Homoeopathic materia medica* is the study of homeopathic remedies which have been tested on human volunteers.

maternal referring to the mother; the quality of being a mother.

Maternal and Child Health (MCH) facilities and programmes organized to provide health and social services to mothers and children.

maternal antibodies antibodies transferred from the mother to the fetus across the placenta. Babies are born with some immunity.

maternal death the death of the mother during the reproductive cycle.

maternal–infant bonding the complex process by which the mother and child become emotionally attached. It starts in the period before delivery and may take some time to accomplish. Interaction and responsiveness are shared.

maternal mortality rate the number of deaths in the reproductive cycle per 100 000 live and stillbirths. The Confidential Enquiry into Maternal Deaths is published triennially and gives detail of deaths anonymously.

maternity motherhood.

Maternity Alliance a charity which campaigns for improvements in maternity services. It provides education, support, research and publications.

maternity allowance the benefit given to pregnant women when they stop work on condition that they have paid National Insurance contributions for at least 26 out of the 66 weeks before which the baby is expected to be born. The payment is made for 18 weeks. There is a higher rate or a lower rate paid depending on the salary of the woman.

Maternity Services Liaison Committee a local committee set up to enable communication between consumers and providers (midwives, managers, obstetricians, paediatricians and anaesthetists) of maternity services.

matrix an intercellular substance, the basic building block from which a specific organ or kind of tissue develops.

Matthews–Duncan expulsion of the placenta the maternal surface of the placenta is seen first at the vulva during the third stage of labour (*see* Figure 86). The cause may be a lower lying placenta. (*Compare* Schultze expulsion.)

maturation the process by which the greatest possible amount of development is achieved.

mature fully developed, having ripened, reached full potential.

Mauriceau–Smellie–Veit manoeuvre a method of delivering the aftercoming head

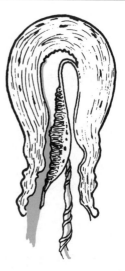

■ **Figure 86** Matthews–Duncan expulsion of the placenta

when a vaginal breech delivery is occurring. Flexion of the head is promoted and jaw and shoulder traction is applied by the hands of the operator who has one hand over the shoulders with the middle finger on the occiput, and the other hand over the chest with the middle finger on the jaw bone (*see* Figure 87).

Maxolon® (metoclopramide) drug given orally or intramuscularly to treat nausea.

mean one form of measurement of central tendency; all the values in a group are added together and divided by the number of values to reach the mean average.

measles a highly infectious disease caused by a virus. Mortality rate is high in some parts of the world. Routine immunization is given after the infant is 1 year old.

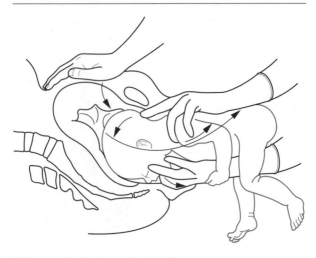

■ **Figure 87** Mauriceau–Smellie–Veit manoeuvre

measles, mumps and rubella vaccine (MMR) an active immunizing agent prescribed to protect the child (or an adult) against these diseases. It is given after the first year of life.

meatus an anatomical passageway opening into or out of an organ.

mechanism of labour a sequence of movements made by the baby as it adapts itself to the changing dimensions of the pelvis during the second stage of labour.

meconium sticky green/black material passed by the baby during the first couple of days after birth. It contains bile pigments, salts, mucus and cells which have collected during pregnancy. It may be passed in utero, possibly as a result of maternal stress or during periods of hypoxia (meconium-stained liquor).

meconium aspiration inhalation of meconium contaminated liquor causing damage to the lining of the lungs.

meconium plug syndrome the meconium becomes very thick and causes the large intestine to be obstructed. The newborn infant will not pass meconium, will have a distended bowel and may vomit.

median 1. situated in the middle or mid-line. 2. a form of measurement of central tendency where a number of values are placed in order (e.g. from least to greatest) and the central one is taken as the median average.

median nerve nerve of the terminal branches of the brachial plexus which extends along the radial parts of the forearm and the hand and supplies muscles and skin. Can be damaged in shoulder dystocia or medically managed breech births with paralysis of the infant's arm.

medical model a traditional approach to treatment in which the practitioner views the human body as a machine, focuses on diagnosis and treatment of a condition or defect within the body and, in the case of pregnancy and birth, assumes normality only in retrospect.

Medical Research Council (MRC) the body responsible for supervising research projects.

Medicines Act 1968 this Act of Parliament established a system for licensing, selling, supplying, controlling and administering of medicines to the public. Midwives are obliged to follow these regulations.

Medicines (Prescription only) Order 1983 schedule 3, parts I and III, gives details of medicines available for practising midwives to use which must be obtained on a doctor's prescription. They include analgesics (pethidine), oxytocics, sedatives and drugs for neonatal resuscitation.

MEDLARS an acronym for Medical Literature Analysis and Retrieval System, a computerized bibliographic system from which the Index Medicus is produced.

MEDLINE an acronym for MEDLARS Online.

medroxyprogesterone acetate (Depo-Provera®) a single dose intramuscular injection of a contraceptive drug which will be effective for 12 weeks.

medulla the central or inside region of an organ. The *medulla oblongata* is the lowest part of the brain at the back just before the spine starts. It controls the vital centres, heart, respiration, etc.

mega- combining form meaning large or as a prefix meaning million, as in megawatt, megavolt, etc.

megaloblastic anaemia an anaemia associated with pregnancy

in which the red blood cells are large and immature and therefore do not bind with oxygen. It is caused by a folic acid deficiency and treated with the same.

megaloblasts large immature red blood cells found in the bone marrow which nevertheless have a nucleus.

meiosis the division of the sex cell into two haploid gametes, the nucleus of each receiving half the number of chromosomes (23).

melanin the black or dark brown pigment which occurs naturally in skin, hair and the iris of the eye. In pregnancy there is an increase in the pigmentation giving rise to the linea nigra, darkened areolas and sometimes chloasma.

membrane a thin tissue covering organs and lining cavities. Frequently responsible for secreting mucus or hormones. Fetal membranes are the amnion and the chorion.

membranes strip a procedure performed during vaginal examination, where a finger is inserted through the external cervical os and gently frees the membranes from the wall of the lower segment of the uterus. This may stimulate the release of oxytocin and commencement of labour.

menadione (SYNONYM menaphthone) a synthetic form of vitamin K. It is water based and usually given by injection.

menarche the onset of menstruation in young girls; the first menstrual period.

Mendel's law the principles of genetic inheritance which indicate how characteristics are passed from one generation to the next.

Mendelson's syndrome an inflammatory response to inhalation of regurgitated gastric juices during the induction of a general anaesthetic. The juices burn the lining of the lungs causing irritation, spasm and oedema. Can occasionally be fatal, but is preventable by the application of cricoid pressure.

meninges the three membranes covering the brain and spinal cord: dura mater, arachnoid mater and pia mater.

meningitis inflammation of the meninges characterized by headaches, stiffness of the neck, irritability, malaise, nausea, vomiting, delirium, pyrexia and tachycardia. Can be fatal.

meningocele a congenital abnormality characterized by a defect in the skull or vertebral column through which the meninges protrude. The sac is filled with cerebrospinal fluid (*see* Figure 88).

meningoencephalocele a hernia-like protrusion of meninges and brain tissue through a defect in the skull.

meningomyelocele a hernia-like protrusion of meninges and spinal cord through a defect in the vertebral column (*see* Figure 89).

menopause the normal, permanent cessation of menstruation.

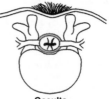

■ **Figure 89**
Meningomyelocele

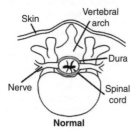

Normal

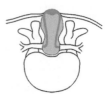

Occulta

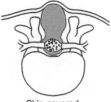

Skin-covered

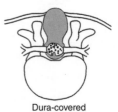

Dura-covered

■ **Figure 88** Meningocele

It signifies the end of the reproductive phase of a woman's life.

menorrhagia unusually heavy bleeding during menstruation.

menorrhoea normal discharge of blood and tissue from the uterus once a month; menstruation.

menostasis impediment in the menstrual flow – discharges cannot escape from the uterus or vagina owing to an occlusion.

menses menstruation.

menstrual referring to menstruation, as in *menstrual period*, the period during the menstrual cycle in which menstruation occurs.

menstrual age the age of an embryo or fetus as it is calculated from the first day of the last normal menstrual period.

menstrual cycle the recurring cycle of changes in the endometrium of the uterus (*see* Figure 90). The decidual layer grows, proliferates, is maintained for several days and then shed at the next period, usually 28 days later. The cycle is controlled by hormones from the pituitary gland and from the

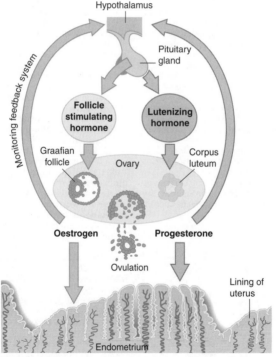

■ **Figure 90** Menstrual cycle

ovaries. The duration and length of the cycle varies greatly among women. This cyclical process begins at the menarche and ends at the menopause.

menstruation (menses, menstrual period) the shedding of blood, cells and other debris from the degenerated deciduas which pass from the non-pregnant uterus through the vagina. It happens at approximately 28-day intervals and lasts about 4–5 days, although there are wide variations in these averages between individual women.

mental pertaining to the mind.

mentoanterior the position of the fetus in the uterus with the chin at the front of the pelvis (*see* Figure 91). Other possible chin positions are mentoposterior and mentolateral.

mentor an experienced practitioner who helps or guides a student or less experienced person.

mentum the chin; used as the denominator in a face presentation of the fetus.

meptazinol (Meptid®) an analgesic drug claimed to cause less respiratory depression than pethidine. May cause nausea and vomiting.

meridian one of the energy lines running throughout the body along which acupuncture points are located in Traditional Chinese Medicine.

mesentery the membranes which line the abdominal cavity and fold over to hold the abdominal organs in place.

mesoderm the layer of cells between the ectoderm and the endoderm in the embryo which will develop into bone, muscle, heart, blood, gonads, kidneys and connective tissue.

mesosalpinx the part of the peritoneum which covers the fallopian tubes.

mesovarium the part of the peritoneum connecting the ovary to the broad ligament.

meta-analysis examination of several research studies on the same topic in order to reach a collective conclusion.

metabolic acidosis an abnormal physiological state in which there is excessive loss of bicarbonate from the body and accumulation of acids in the blood.

metabolism all the processes that take place in living organisms resulting in growth, energy, elimination, and other bodily functions as they relate to the use of nutrients in the blood after absorption from the gut.

metatarsum the part of the foot between ankle and toes where there are five metatarsals.

methadone hydrochloride a synthetic compound with effects similar to that of morphine and heroin. Prescribed in pregnancy to drug addicts as a maintenance drug.

methyldopa a drug used to treat high blood pressure present before pregnancy. It crosses the placental barrier.

metralgia tenderness or pain in the uterus.

metric system a decimalized system of measurement based on kilograms, metres and litres rather than pounds, feet and pints.

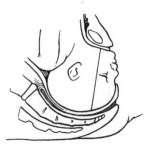

■ **Figure 91** Mentoanterior

metritis inflammation of the walls of the uterus, may be *endometritis* or *parametritis*.

metropathia haemorrhagica excessive painless menstrual and intermenstrual bleeding accompanied by lack of ovulation.

metroplasty surgical operation to repair the uterus.

metrorrhagia bleeding from the uterus that is not the menstrual period.

metrostaxis persistent slight bleeding from the uterus.

micro- combining form meaning very small.

microbe an organism too small to see with the naked eye. Can be seen with a microscope.

microcephaly abnormal smallness of the head. Such babies are mentally subnormal.

microgenitalism abnormal smallness of the external reproductive organs.

micrognathia abnormal smallness of the lower jaw bone; receding chin. Associated with Pierre Robin syndrome.

Microgynon 30® a contraceptive pill containing oestrogen and progesterone.

micron one millionth part of a meter – a micrometre.

Micronor® a contraceptive pill containing only progesterone, used by breastfeeding mothers and those with sensitivity to oestrogen or a history of thrombosis.

micro-organism a tiny living cell too small to be seen with the human eye.

microphage a neutrophil capable of ingesting small organisms such as bacteria.

micturition passing of urine.

MIDIRS Midwives Information and Resource Service.

mid-stream urine, mid-stream catch urine specimen a collection of urine obtained after the genitalia have been cleansed, the stream started, the mid-section saved and voiding completed in the toilet. It should be freer from contamination than a standard urine sample.

midwife traditionally, a woman who was with other women during childbirth. According to the International Confederation of Midwives and the International Federation of Gynaecologists and Obstetricians, following the definition developed by the World Health Organization, a midwife is 'a person who, having been regularly admitted to a midwifery education programme, duly recognized in the country in which it is located, has successfully completed the prescribed course of studies in midwifery and has acquired the requisite qualifications to be registered and/or legally licensed to practise midwifery. She (or he) must be able to give the necessary supervision, care and advice to women during pregnancy, labour and the postpartum period, to conduct deliveries on her (his) own responsibility and to care for the newborn and the infant. The care includes preventative measures, the detection of abnormal conditions in mother and child, the procurement of medical assistance and the execution of emergency measures in the absence of medical help. She (or he) has an important task in health counselling and health education, not only for the patients [sic], but also within the family and the community. The work should involve antenatal education and preparation for parenthood and extends to certain areas of gynaecology, family planning and childcare. She (or he) may practise in hospitals, clinics, health units, domiciliary conditions or in any other service.' This definition is considered contentious by some, as it does not include traditional midwives who practise in some parts of the world or those midwives who did not learn through institutional programmes.

midwifery the art and science concerned with caring for women and their families during normal pregnancy, labour and the postnatal period.

Midwives Acts parliamentary legislation to regulate the practice of midwives. Acts were passed in 1902, 1918, 1926 and 1936. These were consolidated in the Midwives Act 1951 and all came under the umbrella of the Nurses, Midwives and Health Visitors Acts of 1979 and 1992 when a new structure for regulation of these professions was put in place.

Midwives Code of Practice a code set out by the Nursing and Midwifery Council (NMC). It contains guidance on issues relating to midwifery practice in the UK. Although it is guidance rather than a legal obligation, failure to comply with the code could be used as evidence against a midwife were she to be referred to the disciplinary committee of the NMC.

Midwives Rules legislation put in place by the Nursing and Midwifery Council (NMC) with which all midwives must comply. These rules are part of the regulation of midwifery and relate to education, practice and supervision of midwives by the local supervising authority.

milia neonatorum tiny cysts found on the face or trunk of the newborn. They wash off over the next few days.

military attitude used to describe the fetal head which is neither flexed or deflexed.

milk the bodily fluid secreted by the mammary glands.

milk ejection reflex (SYNONYM 'let-down' reflex) as the baby starts sucking at the breast the neurohormonal arch is stimulated and oxytocin is released from the posterior aspect of the pituitary gland. It causes the myoepithelial cells to contract forcing the milk towards the nipple.

milk fever the mild pyrexia occurring on postnatal days 4 and 5 as lactation commences.

milli- a prefix meaning one-thousandth of the whole, e.g. milligram (mg), millilitre (ml), millimetre (mm).

Milton a brand of antiseptic containing 1% solution of sodium hypochlorite. It must be diluted to sterilize babies' feeding utensils and bottles.

miscarriage (SYNONYM abortion) the spontaneous loss from the uterus of a baby before the 24th week of gestation. It may be loss altogether (*complete abortion*) or in part (*incomplete abortion*) or the fetus may die and be retained (*missed abortion*).

missed abortion death but not expulsion of the fetus before 24th week of gestation. Signs of pregnancy diminish.

Misuse of Drugs Act 1971 legislation to control the possession and supply of certain drugs deemed to be liable to misuse or addiction. These include Omnopon®, pethidine, cocaine, morphine and diamorphine.

mitosis the way in which cells reproduce themselves. The nucleus divides and so does each chromosome so that two identical cells are produced.

mitteleschmerz pain between menstrual periods; thought to originate in the reproductive organs and to coincide with ovulation.

mobile epidural an epidural catheter is inserted and low strength bupivacaine is put into the epidural space in such a way that sensory nerves are bathed and blocked but not motor nerves, allowing the woman to retain movement of her lower limbs and control of her bladder.

mode a measurement of central tendency which comprises the value or term which occurs more frequently than any other value or term.

modified milk cows' milk in which the ratios of fat and protein have been changed to more closely resemble those of human milk.

module a short programme of study in a specific area designed to meet a limited number of objectives. Modules are awarded credit towards a higher qualification.

Mogadon® (nitrazepam) a drug used as night sedation.

molar pregnancy a hydatidiform mole develops after conception instead of a fetus. All the signs of pregnancy are severely exaggerated. Removal under anaesthetic is usually required.

mole 1. in dermatology, a small area of skin which is deeply pigmented. 2. in obstetrics, a hydatidiform mole. 3. in science, a unit of measure of a substance.

molecular genetics the branch of genetic study which focuses on the chemical transmission of information, i.e. deoxyribonucleic acid (DNA).

molecule the smallest particle of a substance or fluid. Molecules are different sizes depending on the material of which they form a part. Molecules contain atoms.

Mongolian blue spot a smooth brown or greyish area of skin present at birth. It is due to an excess of melanocytes in one particular area, frequently over the sacrum. They fade or disappear during childhood.

mongolism old term for Down's syndrome.

monitrice a labour coach, usually a person with special training in the Lamaze method of childbirth.

monoamine oxidase inhibitors (MAO) a group of drugs used to treat depression.

monosaccharide the simplest form of sugar.

monotrophy a mother's ability to bond with only one child of twins at a time. This may happen if one infant has remained in a special care unit after discharge of its sibling.

monozygote referring to, or developed from, a single fertilized cell. The cell divides and identical twins can develop (*see* Figure 92).

mons veneris the area over the symphysis pubis which is covered with hair.

Montgomery's glands, Montgomery's tubercles sebaceous glands around the nipples which secrete material which lubricates and protects the nipple from infection and trauma during breastfeeding.

morbid diseased, physically or mentally.

morbidity the condition of being diseased.

morbidity rate the number of cases of a particular disease occurring in a year in a specific number of the population. It may be calculated on the basis of age group, live or stillbirth, sex, or other population unit.

'morning after' pill a large dose of oestrogen given orally within 72 hours of unprotected sexual intercourse to prevent a conception occurring.

morning sickness the feeling of nausea and occasional vomiting sometimes associated with

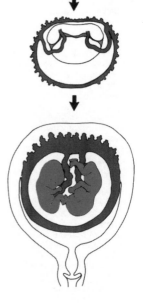
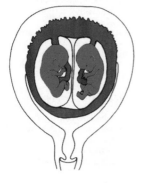

(a) Separate amnions; common chorion and placenta

(b) Common amnion, chorion, and placenta

▉ Figure 92 Monozygote twins

early pregnancy. It may happen at any time of day.

Moro reflex the response of a healthy newborn baby to a sudden noise or the falling back of its head. The arms swing out and return to a central position in a series of small jerks.

morphine sulphate a powerful drug made from opium given on a doctor's prescription to relieve severe pain. It may cause depression of the respiratory centre in the brain.

mortality rate (SYNONYM death rate) the number of deaths in a given population – e.g. *maternal, neonatal* or *infant mortality rate.*

morula the fertilized ovum at 4 days old, when cell division has occurred and it resembles a small mulberry.

motor nerves the nerves through which impulses pass from the spinal cord to muscles instructing them to move in a desired manner.

moulding a process of alteration of the shape and size of the fetal head during its passage through the maternal pelvis as it accommodates itself to the

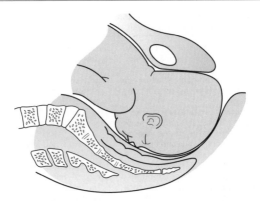

■ **Figure 93** Moulding

bony structure while protecting the brain (*see* Figure 93). The soft sutures between the bones allow overriding of the bones and this can be felt on vaginal examination.

mouth-to-mouth resuscitation a procedure in which the mouth of a breathing person covers that of a non-breathing person and air is forcibly blown into the non-breathing lungs to maintain oxygenation and so maintain the person's life.

movements *fetal movements* start as twitches and progress to full limb and breathing movements. The mother is usually not aware of them until approximately 19 weeks' gestation.

mucoid describes a body fluid as being thick and like egg white.

mucopurulent containing mucus which is infected and yellowed by the presence of pus.

mucosa (SYNONYM mucous membrane) a membrane which produces mucus.

mucous referring to or secreting mucus.

mucous membrane (SYNONYM mucosa) a thin sheet of tissue which covers or lines cavities, organs and canals in the body. Its function is to protect structures, secrete mucus to prevent friction and allow movement, and absorb water salts and other substances (including drugs).

mucus a clear, thick fluid secreted by the body to reduce friction between adjacent tissues.

mucus plug the operculum is the plug of mucus which fills the cervical canal during pregnancy and is shed as the 'show' at the commencement of cervical dilation in labour. Entry of sperm and some microorganisms is prevented.

müllerian ducts the ducts present in early fetal life which in females will fuse to become the vagina, uterus and fallopian tubes. Most of the ducts will disappear in the male fetus.

multicultural refers to a community in which people from many different cultures and ethnic backgrounds live.

multidisciplinary team a group of people each trained in a specific and different branch of health care who work together to achieve common objectives.

multifactorial a situation in which many factors will be relevant and influence the result.

multigravida a pregnant woman who has had at least one previous pregnancy.

multipara a woman who has given birth to more than one infant.

multiple pregnancy a pregnancy in which there is more than one fetus in the uterus. Twins occur spontaneously in approximately 1:80 pregnancies. Triplet and higher-order pregnancies are less common.

multiple sclerosis a progressive disease in which nerves become demyelinated giving rise to strange sensations and symptoms of ataxia, tremor and urogenital disturbances among others.

mumps a communicable disease caused by a virus infecting the parotid glands (saliva-producing glands in the mouth). Rarely seen today as immunization is offered during the second year of life.

murmur a sound heard periodically on auscultation, usually of cardiac or vascular origin. It is deemed pathological.

muscle a specialized group of cells with the ability to contract and relax. The cells may be arranged in bundles and pairs will work opposite each other in the major limbs. They may be arranged in circular formation and called sphincters, e.g. the anus and the iris, or they may be arranged in sheets and not be under the control of the central nervous system, as in the intestines.

muscular dystrophy a genetic disease in which generalized muscle wasting occurs resulting in crippling. *Duchenne muscular dystrophy* is a sex-linked recessive disease in which a woman carries the disease and will pass it on the her daughters, who may become carriers, or her sons, one in two of whom will have the disease. It can now be detected antenatally by DNA studies.

Nn

Naboth's cysts (nabothian cysts) small cysts on the cervix caused by blockage of the entrance to the nabothian glands.

nabothian glands mucous secreting glands on the uterine cervix.

NAD acronym meaning nothing abnormal detected.

Nägele's pelvis a pelvis in which one of the sacral ala fails to develop causing the pelvis to be abnormally shaped making a normal delivery difficult.

Nägele's rule a method of calculating the expected date of delivery of the fetus. Subtract 3 months from the date of the last normal menstrual period and add a year and 7 days, or add 7 days and 9 months to the date of the last normal menstrual period. This system presumes a 28-day menstrual cycle and has been shown to be less than optimally accurate.

naevus (nevus) a birthmark caused by a small area of dilated capillary blood vessels on the skin.

nalidixic acid an antibacterial drug which may be prescribed to treat urinary tract infections (UTI).

naloxone (Narcan®) the drug used as an antidote to pethidine-like drugs if the mother has received a narcotic type drug in labour and it is thought likely that the newborn will have respiratory depression as a result. This drug may be offered to the mother intravenously in the second stage of labour, or to the newborn after birth to reverse the depressant effect.

named midwife the midwife who is primarily working with a woman; ideally in such a way that a therapeutic relationship develops. The midwife may offer continuity of carer to the woman or coordinate care from other professionals if required.

nano- prefix meaning one thousand millionth, e.g. *nanogram* (ng).

napkin rash (nappy rash) occurs on the nappy area. There are red areas, which may have tiny raised patches resembling blisters. It can be caused by the skin being covered or enclosed, ammonia in the urine being in contact with the skin for a long time, or by fungal infection.

Narcan® *see* naloxone.

narco- combining form meaning stupor.

narcotic a drug which lowers the conscious level to produce insensibility or stupor.

narcotic addict a person in the habit of taking narcotic drugs, and who may obtain them illegally or without a prescription in order to induce a state of changed consciousness.

narcotic antagonist a drug used to reverse the respiratory depressing effect of narcotic drugs (nalorphine, levallorphan, naloxone).

nares the nostrils.

nasal relating to the nose.

nasogastric tube a thin, soft latex tube passed into the stomach via the nose of the neonate in order to assess patency of the oesophagus, to aspirate mucus, or to feed.

nasopharynx that part of the nose above the soft palate of the mouth.

natal referring to birth.

National Childbirth Trust (NCT) a charity which runs childbirth education sessions, provides breastfeeding support and sets up postnatal support groups. The NCT also publishes a magazine and works on providing accurate information to consumers. Teachers are trained to diploma level.

National Health Service (NHS) system set up in 1948 by the UK government to allow health care access to all citizens. It is now arranged in eight regions containing more than 80 health authorities. These authorities are divided into 450 NHS trusts. The trusts are run at local level in an attempt to assess and meet local needs. They have a set budget for which they are accountable.

natural childbirth a philosophy which encourages giving birth without routine medical intervention.

natural family planning controlling fertility without resort to medication or mechanical devices, the principle being to avoid unprotected intercourse around the time of ovulation as predicted by measuring basal temperature, checking physical signs such as cervical position and quality of mucus or calculating likely ovulation date from data on previous cycles.

nausea the sensation of wanting to be sick. Nausea and vomiting is one of the earliest signs of pregnancy. It is also frequently a side-effect of medication.

navel the umbilicus or belly button.

necro- combining form meaning death.

necrosis death of a small mass of tissue within a larger mass as a result of injury or infection.

necrotic affected by necrosis.

necrotizing enterocolitis inflammation of the gut wall of a neonate as a result of infection. Recognized by acute abdominal pain, blood in the stools and vomiting, the condition may lead to septicaemia and is life-threatening.

needlestick injury accidental damage to the skin of a person by a needle which has previously been used to treat another person. The risk of cross-infection with human immunodeficiency virus or hepatitis is potentially great. Rigorous attention to safe disposal of needles is required of all health care staff.

negligence a deficiency in the care delivered as compared to that delivered by a reasonable person in the same circumstances. If damage results it is a professional offence and will be investigated and disciplined within the profession as authorized by legislation. Victims of negligence may proceed to law to claim compensation.

neo- combining form meaning new, young.

neomycin a drug used to treat infections.

neonatal pertaining to the newborn infant from birth up to 4 weeks of age.

Neonatal Behavioural Assessment Scale (NBAS) a means of assessing an infant's condition, alertness, motor function, irritability, consolability and interaction with people.

neonatal death (NND) death of an infant within the first 4 weeks of life.

neonatal mortality rate the number of deaths among infants up to 4 weeks of age, per 1000 live births occurring within 1 year.

neonatal period the time from birth until 28 days of age when the infant is at greatest risk of infection and failure to thrive.

neonatal thermoregulation newborn babies are incapable of achieving a balance of heat loss and heat retention. They lose heat through conduction, radiation, evaporation and convection. Care is required to minimize heat loss by drying and covering the baby (especially the head) quickly after birth.

neonatal unit an area of a hospital especially resourced and staffed to meet the needs of babies born unwell, premature, or with injuries and abnormalities.

neonate an infant during its first 28 days of life.

neonatology the study, treatment and care of neonates.

Nepenthe® (morphine) strong analgesic.

nephritis inflammation of a kidney. It is usually secondary to an infection somewhere else in the body.

nephron a unit of the kidney's substance which is involved in filtration of blood.

nerve a fibre which carries messages between the brain and the different parts of the body.

nerve block disruption of the neural pathway by drugs. Sensation of pain is interrupted by nerves being bathed in a drug such as bupivacaine. Otherwise known as epidural analgesia.

nervous anxious, worried, slightly afraid.

nervous system the channels supplying the whole body which transmit to the brain (control centre) information about the environment. The channels contain nerves (peripheral nerves) which enter and leave the spinal cord through which their information is relayed to the brain.

network socially and professionally, a range of people with whom one has some things in common and from whom one could seek help and advice if required.

neural tube defect (NTD) when the bones do not grow over the spinal column completely during early fetal development thereby allowing exposure or protrusion of part of the central nervous system, as in open or occult spina bifida.

neuritis inflammation of a nerve.

neurohormonal a harmonic relationship exists between sensory and endocrine pathways. Hormones from the endocrine system react and interact with the nervous system. Stimulation from the nervous system produces an effect, for example the 'let-down' reflex during lactation or contractions during labour.

neuromotor referring to the working of nerves and muscles.

neuromuscular the nerves and muscles work together to achieve a desired state.

neuromuscular harmony different muscles behave differently but their behaviour is synchronized by the nervous system.

neuron, neurone a single nerve cell.

neurosis a condition characterized by emotional instability. The psychological mood swings dramatically with small provocation.

neurotic prone to severe anxiety which causes changes of behaviour.

neutral in chemistry, neither acid nor alkaline.

neutrophil a type of white blood cell or leukocyte.

Neville Barnes forceps two curved instruments which are

applied to grip the unborn baby's head during the latter part of the second stage of labour. Traction is then applied and delivery of the fetal head is achieved – a 'lift out'.

newborn the name given to the baby after complete expulsion from its mother.

niacin part of the vitamin B complex – an essential nutrient in the diet required for healthy skin, gastrointestinal tract and nervous system and the manufacture of sex hormones.

nicotine the toxic substance found in tobacco and now known to damage health and embryonic development.

nipple the pigmented area in the centre of the breast which may or may not protrude (*see* types of nipples and Figure 140, below). The lactiferous ducts (18) have openings in the nipple through which secretions (milk) leave the breast.

nipple shield a concave, nipple-shaped latex cap which is applied over the nipple to protect the tissue from trauma during sucking.

nitrazepam (Mogadon®) a drug used at night to induce sleep.

nitrogen a gaseous element required for the formation of all protein substances.

nitrous oxide a gas which, combined with O_2 in a 50:50 mix, can be inhaled as a mild analgesic in labour.

nocturia passing urine during the night; waking up to urinate.

nocturnal referring to occurrences during the night.

node a small rounded mass which can be palpated.

non-absorbable surgical suture material used to repair a surgical wound such as a perineal tear or episiotomy, which will be dissolved or ingested by enzymes in the tissues.

non-accidental injury damage occurring to the body by deliberate intention of another person. The victim is usually a child.

non-invasive procedure diagnosis or treatment given without the need to penetrate tissues of the body.

non-shivering thermogenesis the natural method for enabling the newborn to maintain its body heat by increasing its metabolic rate and burning stored brown fat.

normotensive having normal blood pressure.

notifiable disease any of a number of conditions the occurrence of which must be made known to the director of public health of the health authority because they can be easily transmitted to other members of the community. They include: infective jaundice, TB, whooping cough, measles, diphtheria and ophthalmia neonatorum.

notification a legal obligation to inform authority representatives. The midwife must notify her intention to practise midwifery to the health authority in her geographical locality.

notification of birth the registrar must be informed of the birth of a baby so that a birth certificate can be issued and population statistics can be compiled.

nucha the nape (lower posterior aspect) of the neck.

nuchal relating to the nape of the neck.

nuchal cord an umbilical cord that is wound around the neck of the fetus during birth.

nuchal fold layer of skin and underlying fat over the back of the neck which can be scanned by ultrasound at an early stage of gestation to measure the thickness (*see* Figure 94). A thickened nuchal fold suggests

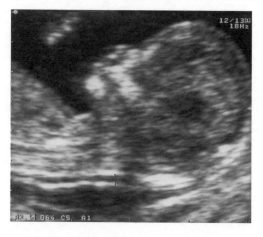

■ **Figure 94** Nuchal fold scan

that further tests should be performed to investigate the possibility of the fetus having Down's syndrome.

nuclear family a small number of closely, usually biologically, related people living together – mother, father and children.

nucleic acid one of a group of long chain proteins found in cells. There are two types: deoxyribonucleic acid (DNA) and ribonucleic acid (RNA).

nucleus the central structure in each cell which contains its genes and controls its behaviour.

nullipara a woman who has not given birth to a live infant.

numbness lack or loss of sensation or feeling.

nurse 1. to breastfeed. 2. a person who has been trained and assessed as being capable of carrying out the duty of care and support necessary to promote health, restore health, and ensure the comfort and well-being of others who need such assistance.

nursery a place where infants and young children are cared for. The local authority registers, supervises and provides nurseries for children under 5 years of age.

Nurses, Midwives and Health Visitors Acts 1979 and 1992 these Acts of Parliament combined the activities of previous individual professional boards under one code of conduct, regulated by the United Kingdom Central Council of Nursing, Midwifery and Health Visiting (UKCC) and having a national board in each country. The UKCC has been replaced by the Nursing and Midwifery Council (NMC).

Nursing and Midwifery Council (NMC) the statutory regulatory authority responsible for registration, training standards, conduct enforced through the Midwives Rules and Code of Practice and discipline of midwives, nurses and health visitors. It investigates malpractice and misconduct. It maintains a public register of people eligible to practise.

nursing process a systematic method of delivering individualized care based on four stages: assessment, planning, implementation and evaluation.

nurture to feed, rear, foster, care for and enable the social development of children.

nutrition the process by which the body takes in and uses food to perform its functions, remain healthy and reproduce.

nymphomania a psychosexual disorder in women characterized by an insatiable desire for sexual intercourse.

nystatin a drug used to treat infections, especially of a fungal nature, e.g. candidiasis. It can be applied topically, orally or vaginally.

Oo

O₂ a clear, colourless gas found in the atmosphere at 21% concentration. It is absorbed into the blood via the lungs and is essential for all bodily activities.

OA *see* occipitoanterior.

obese describes someone with a normal sized skeleton but with a larger than normal amount of soft tissue, causing the body mass index (BMI) to be high.

obesity an excess of fat cells, mainly in the subcutaneous tissue. Body weight is 20% above the desired weight for age, sex and height.

objective 1. of a mind or minds, independent. 2. being evident to other people; measurable. 3. not influenced by personal feelings.

oblique at a slant, not horizontal or vertical.

oblique presentation where the long axis of the fetus (spine) is lying oblique or slanted in relation to the long axis (spine) of the mother.

observation something which is seen or noticed.

obsession a recurrent thought, idea or impulse to act, not necessarily based on logical thinking, which the person feels unable to control and which disturbs the person's mental equilibrium.

obstetric forceps surgical instruments with handles attached to a blunt blade used to surround and apply traction to the fetal head in order to achieve delivery.

obstetrician a doctor who has received additional training in pathological conditions which

may occur in pregnancy, childbirth and the puerperium.

obstetrics the branch of medicine concerned with caring for women in pregnancy, childbirth and the puerperium.

obstructed labour an arrest or interruption to the process of giving birth due to a restriction in the birth canal (*see* Figure 95).

obturator a device applied to block a space, canal or passage.

occipital referring to the region at the back of the head, just above the neck.

occipital bone the cup-like bone at the back of the skull marked by a large opening called the foramen magnum.

occipitoanterior (OA) relationship of the fetal head within

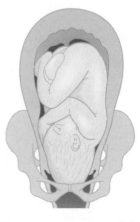

■ **Figure 95** Obstructed labour

the maternal pelvis. The back of the fetal head is to the front of the maternal pelvis.

occipitobregmatic diameter on the fetal skull taken from below the occipital protrusion to the anterior fontanelle. In the average term baby it is approximately 10.5 cm. When measured from below the occiput it is the suboccipitobregmatic diameter and is slightly shorter at 9.5 cm.

occipitofrontal diameter of the partially deflexed fetal skull measured from the occipital protrusion to the forehead. It is 11.5 cm in the average term fetus.

occipitolateral a position of the fetal head in relation to the maternal pelvis where the occipital bone is to the side of the mother's pelvis.

occipitoposterior (OP) a position of the fetal head in relation to the maternal pelvis where the occiput is to the back of the pelvis. This is not ideal for labour as the head will either have a long rotation in order to accommodate the curve of the birth canal or will descend through the birth canal in this position (persistent occipitoposterior position), possibly being born face-to-pubes.

occiput the bone at the back of the fetal head and in particular the central part which protrudes.

occlusive cap used as a method of contraception, it is introduced by the woman via the vagina and is applied so that it completely covers the cervix (*see* Figure 96). Often used with a spermicide.

octigravida a woman who is into her eighth pregnancy.

oedema collection of fluid in the tissues of the body.

oesophageal referring to the oesophagus.

oesophageal atresia a congenital abnormality in which the oesophagus ends in a blind loop before reaching the stomach (*see* Figure 97). It may be suspected in pregnancy by the presence of polyhydramnios and may be seen on ultrasound scan. It may be suspected in the neonate who only takes small amounts of its feed or vomits

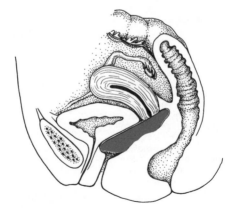

■ **Figure 96** Occlusive cap

undigested milk. Surgical correction is required urgently.

oesophagus the muscular tube which passes food from the back of the throat into the stomach.

oestrogen, estradiol, estriol, estrone hormones from the ovary or placenta which have various effects on the body influencing growth of breast tissue and fat deposits at puberty, development of the lining of the uterus on a monthly cycle ready for implantation of a fertilized ovum, growth of the uterus and breasts in pregnancy, water and electrolyte retention and inhibition of lactation during pregnancy.

oestrogenic a substance (e.g. a plant, herb or pharmaceutical drug) whose effects resemble those of oestrogen.

oestrone *see* oestrogen, estrone.

Office of Population, Censuses and Surveys (OPCS) a government department whose job it is to collect, collate and issue statistics about the population so that planning of services and other research can be carried out.

olfactory referring to the sense of smell.

olfactory nerve the cranial nerve which passes directly from the brain to the nose or nasal area.

oligaemia reduction in the volume of blood.

oligo-, olig- combining form meaning deficiency of, few.

oligohydramnios deficiency in the volume of the amniotic liquor around the fetus in utero. This is associated with congenital abnormalities of the kidney and intrauterine growth restriction.

oligomenorrhoea a slight reduction in menstrual blood loss.

oligospermia a deficiency in the number of sperm in the semen. It is associated with subfertility.

oliguria a deficiency in the volume of urine secreted by the kidney. It is associated with shock and renal failure.

ombudsman an official who investigates complaints about

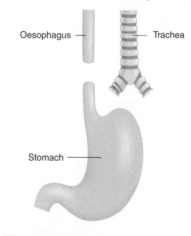

Oesophagus —   — Trachea

Stomach —

■ **Figure 97** Oesophageal atresia

the health services. She passes her evidence to a panel for jurisdiction.

omentum layer of connective tissues which is part of the peritoneum and which holds the stomach alongside its adjacent organs.

Omnopon® (papaveretum) a strong analgesic drug derived from opium which is a controlled drug (*see* controlled drug).

omphalocele a swelling around the umbilicus due to weakness in the muscular sheath over the abdominal cavity.

omphalus the umbilical cord.

o.n. an abbreviation from the Latin being an instruction to give a treatment, usually medicine, at night.

ooblast a primitive cell in the ovary from which the ovum develops and emerges.

oocyte an ovum released but at an immature stage, so a conception is unlikely to be successful.

oophor-, oophoro- combining form meaning ovary.

oophorectomy surgical removal of the ovary.

oophoritis inflammation of the ovary.

oophorosalpingectomy surgical removal of the ovary and the fallopian tube.

OP *see* occipitoposterior.

operation surgical treatment.

operational system a means of recording on computer the care and treatment received by women. It usually covers the entire hospital and/or community services.

operculum the thick plug of mucus found in the cervical canal during pregnancy. It prevents infection entering the uterus and forms the 'show' during the early stages of labour because it emerges as the cervix begins to efface and dilate in response to contractions (*see* Figure 98).

ophthalmia neonatorum an infection in the eyes of a newborn infant with purulent discharge caused by organisms in the vagina entering the eyes as the infant is born. It may be very serious with consequences for the future sight of the infant. Its occurrence must be notified to the director of public health as it may have been caused by a venereal infection.

ophthalmoscope an instrument with a light and a lens used for examining the eyes.

opiate a strong drug derived from opium. It causes sleep or relief from pain. Its use is controlled by statute as it is a drug of addiction (*see* controlled drug).

opinion the advice offered by an expert (a judicial court or a midwifery or medical consultant).

opioid a drug derived from the poppy plant, i.e. morphine with opium like effects on the body. Endorphins and enkephalins produced in the body are thought to be natural opioids.

opium a drug made from unripe capsules of poppies used to manufacture morphine and other very strong drugs.

opportunistic infection an infection which occurs only because the body's defences have been weakened by another recent or current pathological condition.

opsonin a substance which coats bacteria or other cells making it easier for leukocytes to work and destroy them.

optic relating or referring to the eye.

oral refers to the mouth.

oral contraceptive pill a tablet taken by mouth daily which aims to prevent a woman becoming pregnant.

orbit a circular structure, usually referring to the bony cavities in

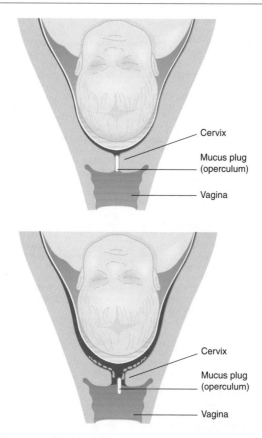

Cervix

Mucus plug
(operculum)

Vagina

Cervix

Mucus plug
(operculum)

Vagina

■ **Figure 98** Operculum

the skull which house and protect the eyeballs.

orbital ridge the upper bony aspect of the orbital cavity, which if felt on vaginal examination indicates a fetus presenting by the brow.

orchi-, orchido- combining form meaning the testes.

orchiopexy an operation in which an undescended testicle is loosened from restraining tissues and brought into the scrotum and attached so that it cannot be retracted.

orchitis inflammation of the testis. May occur as a complication of mumps, syphilis or TB.

organ a group of tissues in the body, usually encapsulated, which have a particular function.

organic a chemical compound containing carbon.

organism a living being, plant or animal.

organogenesis the process during early embryonic life by which the cells of the body migrate to the appropriate sites and become specialized to the function they must perform.

orgasm the climax of masturbation or the sexual act involving strong muscular contractions of the reproductive organs and accompanied in males by ejaculation of semen.

orifice an opening into or out of a cavity or organ.

oropharynx the part of the throat immediately behind the mouth and below the nose.

-orrhaphy word-ending which refers to repair or suturing of something, as in *colporrhaphy*, surgical suturing and repair of the vaginal wall.

orthopaedics the branch of Western medicine concerned with bones and muscles.

Ortolani's test a test done on the hips of newborn infants to detect dislocation.

os 1. bone. 2. mouth or opening. The *cervical os* is the mouth or opening of the uterus. The *external os* is the part of the cervix which forms the opening into the vagina. The *internal os* is the part of the cervix which forms the opening into the uterus.

os innominatum (innominate bone) the three fused bones on either side of the pelvis which form the girdle.

Osiander's sign pulsation of the uterine arteries felt through the walls of the vagina, a sign said to be a presumptive indicator of pregnancy.

osmolality refers to the pressure of a fluid.

osmosis the movement of a pure solvent such as water across a permeable membrane from a solution that has a lower concentration to one of a higher concentration. The movement of fluid continues until the concentration is equal on both sides of the membrane.

osmotic pressure the pressure felt by a semi-permeable membrane which divides a strong solution from a weaker one.

ossification the development of bone by the laying down of calcium.

osteomalacia a condition arising in normally formed bones whereby calcium is lost due to inadequate dietary intake of vitamin D or the minerals calcium and phosphorous. The bones become soft, weak and painful. The equivalent in infants and children is rickets.

osteopathy a form of treatment to correct imbalances in the musculoskeletal system. Diagnosis and correction is by manipulation and massage.

otitis infection of the ear.

-otomy word-ending indicating cutting into.

outlet the route by which exit is achieved.

outlet contracture refers to the pelvis in the rare circumstance where the bones are too close together to allow the fetus to pass through.

output the total amount produced. *Cardiac output* is the amount out of blood the ventricles pump out in a specific time (usually 1 minute).

outreach clinic a clinic away from a main hospital site which may be in a local centre where it is more accessible to the community or a specific group in the population.

ova more than one ovum.

ovarian referring to the ovary.

ovarian cyst a globular sac, fluid or connective tissue filled, on the ovary.

ovarian follicle a small cavity on the ovary which contains a fluid which divides the follicular cells into layers and surrounds an ovum.

ovarian pregnancy a pregnancy which becomes implanted on the wall of or within the ovary. It does not usually survive.

ovariotomy cutting into the ovary. Usually refers to removal of the ovary.

ovary an almond-sized organ found in the broad ligament on either side of the uterus. The ovaries are responsible for producing and maturating an ovum each month and the secretion of the ovarian hormones oestrogen and progesterone. Ovarian activity is governed by the pituitary gland which secretes follicle-stimulating hormone (FSH) and luteinizing hormone (LH). Oestrogen and progesterone form a negative feedback loop in which the pituitary produces less FSH in response to rising levels of oestrogen and less LH in response to rising levels of progesterone. The oestrogen and progesterone cause the lining of the uterus to become thickened and congested with blood in readiness for receipt of a fertilized ovum.

overdose an excessive concentration of a substance in the blood which will cause side-effects and could result in altered consciousness, coma or death.

ovulation the expulsion of a mature ovum from the ovary, a process occurring on average 14 days before the period is due.

ovum the reproductive cell produced by the female body on a regular monthly basis which contains half the chromosomes required to form a conceptus.

oxygen an element found in the form of a gas essential to life. It is clear, colourless and found in a 21% concentration in the atmosphere. It is drawn into the lungs during respiration and crosses the membranes of the alveoli to combine with haemoglobin to form oxyhaemoglobin.

oxyhaemoglobin the substance found in the blood which is haemoglobin and oxygen combined. In this way oxygen can easily be transported around the body and released into cells with a low concentration.

oxytetracycline a powerful antibiotic similar to tetracycline which will destroy a range of bacteria.

oxytocic the name given to a substance which will cause contractions of the uterus.

oxytocin (Syntocinon®) a hormone produced by the posterior pituitary gland which causes contraction of uterine muscle and the lactiferous tubules of the mammary glands, forcing milk towards the nipple. It can now be produced synthetically and is used to induce contractions in the first and second stage of labour and to control haemorrhage in the third stage of labour. It is combined with ergometrine to form a drug called Syntometrine® which may be offered prophylactically to prevent postpartum haemorrhage.

Pp

Po₂ partial pressure of oxygen.

P_aco_2 the part of the total blood gas pressure exerted by carbon dioxide. Normal values are 35–45 mmHg in arterial blood and 40–45 mmHg in venous blood.

P_ao_2 the part of the total blood gas pressure exerted by oxygen. In arterial blood it should be 95–100 mmHg.

pachyonychia congenita a congenital ectodermal defect characterized by thickening of the nails, hard skin on the palms and soles, abnormality of the hair follicles and overgrowth and thickening of the skin of the knees and elbows.

pachyvaginitis an inflammation and thickening of the walls of the vagina.

packed cell volume (PCV) refers to the amount of red cells in a litre of blood. The normal value is around 45%.

packed cells blood cells which have been concentrated down into a smaller volume by centrifuging. Used to treat severe anaemia.

packing material inserted into a wound to ensure slow healing by granulation.

pacifier (SYNONYM dummy) nipple-shaped and made of a rubbery material, it is given to an infant to suck to soothe or comfort it. There is controversy among childcare experts and members of the dental profession over its use.

pad wad of soft material used to apply pressure on the body, act as a cushion or absorb moisture including menstrual blood.

paediatrics the branch of Western medicine concerned with health and disease in children.

paediatrician doctor who specializes in the care of children.

paedophilia an adult with an abnormal interest in sex with children.

pain a sensation caused by stimulation of the sensory nerve endings. It is a subjective sensation with different individual responses and may be perceived as unpleasant and uncomfortable or as a positive bodily message. It is a cardinal symptom in the diagnosis of inflammation, trauma and neoplasm. Pain can be described as mild, dull, acute, generalized, burning, sharp, stabbing or referred. A person in pain may appear distracted, self-focused, narrow focused with altered time perception, to have altered thought processes, and to limit interaction with other people.

pain gate theory see gate control theory of pain (and see Figure 99).

pain in labour this is caused by the uterus contracting and the cervix dilating. The pain is characteristically intermittent, felt in the lower abdomen and sometimes the sacral region, and increases in frequency and intensity. The exact pathology is unknown but theories have been advanced that it may be caused by one or a combination of the following

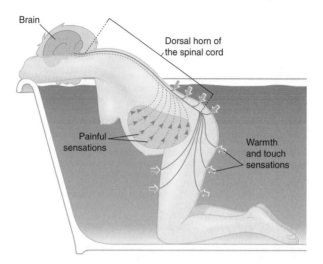

Brain

Dorsal horn of the spinal cord

Painful sensations

Warmth and touch sensations

■ Figure 99 Pain gate theory

features: stretching of the cervix; ischaemia as the uterine contractions reduce the blood flow; pressure on the supporting ligaments.

pain receptor the nerve fibre endings which are found throughout the body. They are stimulated by pressure or heat and their impulses are interpreted by the brain as pain.

palate the roof of the mouth. It is hard at the front and soft at the back. It divides the nose from the mouth. Part of it may be absent due to developmental anomaly and the baby is born with a cleft palate.

pallid pale, skin without colour.

palmar crease the tiny grooves found running across the inside of the clenched hand.

palmar grasp reflex the ability of a newborn to strongly grasp an object which touches the palm of her hand.

palmature a congenital abnormality in which the fingers are webbed one to another.

palpation an examination technique which uses touch. In *abdominal palpation* the abdomen is examined to detect abnormalities, to determine growth of a baby and to assess the lie, presentation, position and engagement of a baby.

palpitation fast beating of the heart which can be detected by physical signs.

palsy an abnormality in which some degree of paralysis is present.

Panadol® (paracetamol) a drug taken in the form of tablets or syrup used to relieve mild pain and reduce fever.

pancreas a large gland found in the upper posterior part of the abdomen which manufactures hormones and enzymes which aid digestion.

pandemic describes an epidemic which is found throughout the population, or worldwide.

pang a sudden or severe spasm of short duration which evokes physical or emotional discomfort.

panic sudden and severe emotional disturbance which results in physical symptoms.

panic attack episode of acute anxiety, apprehension or terror which can cause immobility or strange behaviour.

panting fast, shallow breathing. It may be encouraged by some midwives in the second stage of labour during contractions to slow down emergence of the fetal head through the vulva with the goal of preventing damage to the perineum.

Papanicolaou test (SYNONYMS smear, Pap smear) a screening test in which mucus and cells are scraped off the cervix and examined microscopically to detect cells which may be abnormal or cancerous.

papaveretum (Omnopon®) a drug used in the control of very acute pain. It is a dangerous drug derived from opium, and its use is controlled by legislation.

papilla a small nipple-shaped projection found in different parts of the body.

papilloma a small swelling, non-cancerous, formed of epithelial cells and white in appearance.

PAPP (pregnancy associated plasma proteins) a test which is in development to detect Down's syndrome.

papule small raised area on the skin.

papyraceous like paper. A *fetus papyraceous* is one of twin babies who has died early in pregnancy and has been flattened by the surviving baby to resemble a paper cutout.

para a woman who has borne one or more infants which were more than 24 weeks' gestation. The number of infants is indicated by adding a prefix, e.g. primipara.

parabiotic syndrome transfusion of blood from one twin to another because of vascular anastomoses in the placenta. One twin will be anaemic and one plethoric.

paracentesis a sterile process during which fluid is drawn out of a body cavity. A small incision is made in the skin and a trocar is inserted to allow drainage.

paracervical around the cervix or neck of the uterus.

paracervical block anaesthesia caused by the injection of anaesthetic into the area which contains the nerves. May be used during an instrumental delivery.

paracervix the connective tissue of the pelvic floor extending from the uterine cervix to the side walls of the pelvic cavity.

paracetamol *see* Panadol®.

parachute reflex similar to Moro reflex and startle reflex.

paradigm a particular world view; a pattern used as a model to represent another set of connections, usually of concepts.

paraesthesia a strange sensation described as pins and needles. Experienced as a result of nerve pressure in carpal tunnel syndrome or following an epidural anaesthetic.

paraldehyde a very strong-smelling liquid used to sedate or cause sleep. Can be given by a number of routes and is excreted by the lungs.

paralysis loss of sensation and/or movement caused by anaesthesia, trauma, disease, pressure or poisoning.

paralytic ileus loss of sensation and movement in the intestines, usually temporary and due to surgery or other severe illness. The abdomen is swollen and tender and bowel sounds are absent.

paramedic a person who assists a physician or who has training in emergency medical care; some members of the ambulance service.

parameters a set of values within which normal and abnormal are defined. May also refer to boundaries, borders or limits of normality.

parametritis inflammation of the structures around the uterus.

parametrium the part of the connective tissue covering the uterus which extends sideways to cover the fallopian tubes.

paranoia a condition of the mind in which a person is suspicious of the people around them, who feels that other people are conspiring to harm them in some way, or has delusions or feelings of inferiority or greatness in one aspect of their life.

paranoid subject to feelings of paranoia.

paraphimosis retraction and constriction of the foreskin behind the glans penis making pulling it forward again difficult or impossible.

parasalpingitis inflammation around the fallopian tubes, usually due to infection.

parasite a smaller organism which lives on and relies for its survival on a larger one.

parasympathetic nervous system part of the autonomic nervous system. The parasympathetic nerves slow the heart, stimulate peristalsis, cause tears, bile, insulin, saliva and digestive juices to be produced, dilate peripheral blood vessels, constrict the pupils, oesophagus and bronchioles and cause vasodilatation of the pelvic region allowing congestion of erectile tissue in both sexes.

parathyroid gland four small glands attached to the upper poles of the thyroid gland. They produce parathyroid hormone which helps maintain blood calcium levels, blood clotting, nerve reactivity and cell membrane permeability.

parenchymatous salpingitis inflammation of the functional layer of the fallopian/uterine tube.

parent–infant relationship the relationship – emotional, physical and social – which a child has with its main caregivers.

parentcraft classes a series of meetings of a group of parents with a midwife or other health professional the purpose of which is to discuss topics related to childbirth or child care.

parenteral the giving of drugs or treatment by a route other than the alimentary tract.

parenthood the state whereby an adult becomes responsible for the care and upbringing of a child.

paresis loss of function of motor nerve impulses to muscles but no loss of sensory nerve function.

parietal referring to the top of the head.

parietal bone two of the bones which cover the cranium and pass in a wide band across the top of the head with the anterior fontanelle at the front and the posterior fontanelle at the back.

parity the classification of women according to the number of times they have given birth to a baby of more than 24 weeks' gestation.

parous having borne one or more live children beyond the 24th week of gestation.

paroxysm a sudden increase in the severity of symptoms, fit, seizure, convulsion or spasm.

partial placenta praevia the margin of the placenta is situated over the internal os of the cervix. When the os starts to dilate that part of the placenta may separate causing potentially life-threatening bleeding to the mother and hypoxia to the fetus.

partial pressure the amount of pressure which can be exerted by one gas in a mixture of gases or a liquid. The amount of pressure is dependent on the concentration of that gas in the mixture.

partogram a graphic record of the progress of labour, particularly the dilation of the cervix and descent of the head seen alongside observations of the well-being of the mother and fetus. This record is completed so that abnormalities of progress can be easily identified and action, e.g. augmentation with an oxytocic, initiated.

parturient relating to the process of delivering or giving birth to a baby.

parturition the process of giving birth.

pascal (Pa) an international unit by which pressure may be measured.

passive doing nothing; not active.

passive immunity protection from a disease or infection acquired by a person without action or reaction being required on their part. A fetus obtains this from his mother via the placenta and a neonate via the breast milk.

pasteurization the process of heating up milk to 60°C for 30 minutes so that some of the most harmful bacteria (tuberculosis) will be killed.

pasteurized milk milk which has been treated by pasteurization.

Patau's syndrome congenital abnormality of the chromosomes (trisomy 13), where the infant has misshapen hands, face and feet and mental retardation.

patent open.

patent ductus arteriosus an abnormal condition in which there is a persistence of the fetal circulation, an opening between the aorta and pulmonary artery enabling the larger volume of blood to bypass the lung with reduced oxygen uptake (*see* Figure 100).

paternity refers to the state of having fathered a child.

paternity suit when a mother applies to the courts for money from a man she claims to be the father of her child. In some cases paternity is proved or disproved by DNA testing.

patho-, path-, -pathy combining forms meaning disease.

pathogen an organism which causes disease or infection.

pathologist a person specially trained in the study, detection, and tracking of pathogens.

pathology (1) a branch of science which deals with the nature, cause and progression of disease; (2) the study of disease-causing organisms, usually in a laboratory.

patient person receiving health care; generally used to refer to people who are sick rather than healthy childbearing women.

patient administration system (PAS) a system for the computerization of patient records so that they are held centrally and duplication and error are reduced.

patient-controlled analgesia (PCA) self-regulation of analgesia. Usually reserved for use after major surgery. The analgesia (usually narcotic) is prepared and connected to an i.v. site and syringe pump and the patient depresses a plunger to deliver it. A safety lock-out system prevents overuse/overdose.

Patient's Charter a formal description of some service expectations which can be measured and form a standard

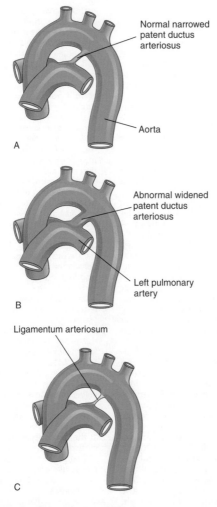

Normal narrowed patent ductus arteriosus

Aorta

A

Abnormal widened patent ductus arteriosus

Left pulmonary artery

B

Ligamentum arteriosum

C

■ **Figure 100** Patent ductus arteriosus

for care. The charter states what patients should expect and the responsibilities of providers of health care and health care staff for the welfare of patients and their families. Maternity services have a charter based on the Changing Childbirth Report.
patulous referring to something that is open or spread apart.

May refer to the cervical os in the postnatal period.

Pawlik's grip a method of assessing engagement of the presenting part during pregnancy. The index finger and thumb of one hand are applied just above the symphysis pubis and the presenting part is ballotted. It can be painful for the mother and is not recommended in practice.

Pco₂ the pressure of carbon dioxide in the blood. Normally it is 40 mmHg.

PCV (packed cell volume) refers to the amount of red blood cells in a litre of blood.

pectoral referring to the breast or chest, or the large muscles over the breast and thorax – pectoralis major and minor.

pedigree line of descent through the generations of a family. Some diseases can be traced from one generation to another.

PEEP (positive end expiratory pressure) used to treat neonates with immature lungs. It keeps the alveoli and dead air spaces inflated and prevents collapse on expiration.

peer review a means of evaluating the professional practice of a colleague of equal status according to preset standards, and done as part of an audit of the service.

pelvic referring to the pelvis.

pelvic bones the innominate bones (fusion of the ilium, ischium and pubis) which form the pelvic girdle along with the sacrum and symphysis pubis.

pelvic brim the part of the pelvis which the baby enters before or during labour. The brim is bordered by the symphysis pubis, superior ascending ramus, sacroiliac joints, iliopectineal lines, ala and sacral promontory.

pelvic congestion increase in blood volume supplying the organs in the pelvis; found in early pregnancy and just before a woman's period is due.

pelvic examination an examination performed by inserting two fingers into the vagina to feel the size and shape of the pelvis, position and condition of the organs.

pelvic floor the two layers of muscles lying across the outlet of the pelvic girdle.

pelvic floor exercises exercises done to tighten and tone the muscles of the pelvic floor in order to restore their function after childbirth.

pelvic haematoma extravascular collection of blood; if sufficiently large it may cause pain and pressure sensations.

pelvic inflammatory disease (PID) severe illness originating from infection of the genital tract which has spread to the pelvic reproductive organs. Can lead to infertility.

pelvic inlet the first area of the bony pelvis through which a fetus will pass during birth (*see* Figure 101).

pelvic outlet the last area of the pelvis through which the fetus will pass during birth (*see* Figure 101).

pelvimeter callipers used to measure the diameters of the pelvis and assess its capacity to accommodate the fetus.

pelvis the bony girdle formed by the pelvic bones and closed at the lower aspect by the pelvic floor muscles (*see* Figure 102). The organs contained within the girdle are bowel, rectum, bladder, uterus, fallopian tubes and ovaries.

pendulous hanging down loosely, dangling.

pendulous abdomen the pregnant abdomen hangs down when the abdominal wall muscles are weakened by a large number of previous pregnancies or large babies.

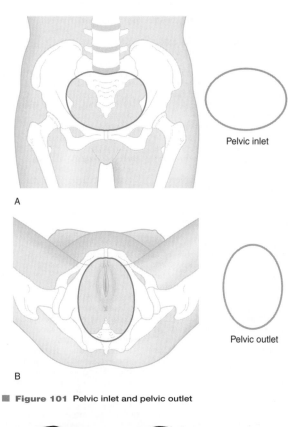

A

B

■ Figure 101 Pelvic inlet and pelvic outlet

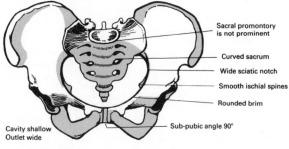

Sacral promontory
is not prominent

Curved sacrum

Wide sciatic notch

Smooth ischial spines

Rounded brim

Cavity shallow
Outlet wide

Sub-pubic angle 90°

■ Figure 102 Pelvis

penetrate to enter, maybe with difficulty.

penicillin an antibiotic made from cultures of species of the fungus *Penicillium.*

penis male organ made of erectile tissue and through which passes the urethra for the transport of urine and spermatozoa.

pentazocine hydrochloride (Fortral®) a narcotic analgesic drug used to relieve severe pain.

peptic referring to the stomach or digestive enzymes.

peptide a chain of molecules made up of amino acids (digested proteins).

per by, around, near to, enclosing.

per vaginam through the vagina.

percentile a term used in statistics. One percentile is a 100th part of the whole. The 80th percentile means that 80% of the population being studied fall below a known or specified range and 20% above. *Percentile charts* are used to show the likely birth weight of babies at different gestations.

percussion tapping a part of the body and listening for vibrations to diagnose boundaries, size or contents of a body cavity.

perforate to make a hole in, or pierce.

performance indicators a means of measuring quality of care by a professional. May be done as part of a process of clinical auditing.

peri- prefix meaning around about an organ (e.g. *perimetric,* relating to the *perimetrium*) or time period (e.g. *perinatal,* around the time of birth; *perimenopausal,* around the time of menopause).

pericranium the membrane of connective tissue which surrounds or lines the inside of the skull bones.

perimetrium the membranes around the outside of the uterus.

perinatal around the time or process of birth.

perinatal death the death of a fetus around the time of birth or an infant within the first week of life. This includes stillbirths and early neonatal deaths.

perinatal mortality the statistical expression of combined deaths per 1000 live births.

perinatologist a doctor who specializes in the care of disorders occurring in mother and infant during pregnancy and childbirth.

perineal refers to the perineum. Because of its position the perineum is vulnerable to trauma and infection during childbirth and it may need repair.

perineal care refers to the need to keep the perineum clean and the performance of exercises to restore function.

perineorrhaphy a surgical procedure in which the perineum is cleaned and repaired.

perineum the area of skin and muscle between the anus and the vagina which supports the internal organs of the pelvic cavity (*see* Figure 103) and which stretches to allow the baby to be born.

period an interval of time. In everyday language the term is used to describe the menses or menstrual period, the monthly loss of blood from the uterus as part of the menstrual cycle.

periodic apnoea of the newborn irregular pattern of breathing with rapid respiration followed by a period of apnoea present in the normal full-term infant.

peripheral at the extremities or ends, usually meaning the limbs.

peripheral resistance the failure of the blood vessels

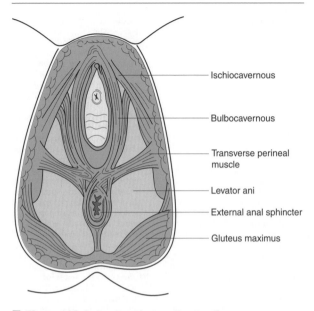

Ischiocavernous

Bulbocavernous

Transverse perineal muscle

Levator ani

External anal sphincter

Gluteus maximus

■ **Figure 103** Perineum and supporting muscles

furthest from the heart to yield to its contractile forces.

periphery the parts on the boundaries.

peristalsis the rhythmic muscular contractions which pass along a tube causing material in the tube to be pushed through.

peritoneum two sheets of membranes, the parietal peritoneum and the visceral peritoneum, the first of which lines the internal abdomen and the other the intestines. The two sheets glide over each other and are lubricated by a little serous fluid.

peritonitis inflammation of the sheets of membrane (peritoneum) lining the abdominal cavity.

periventricular haemorrhage a bleed occurring into the cavities or around the ventricles within the brain. It occurs in preterm babies and can cause death. It is also an assumed cause of cerebral palsy.

permeable a membrane or sheet of tissue through which fluids can pass.

pernicious very harmful or destructive.

pernicious anaemia an anaemia due to the failure of the gastric juices to produce an intrinsic factor which allows absorption of vitamin B_{12}.

perodactyly congenital deformity of the fingers or toes including absence of some digits.

peropus congenital deformity of the feet.

persistent mentoposterior position this describes the position of the baby in the uterus where the head is fully extended and the face is presenting as the part likely to be delivered first. The chin is the denominator and is in the posterior quadrant of the pelvis. It does not rotate during labour. Vaginal delivery is not always possible.

persistent occipitoposterior position describes the position of the fetus in the uterus where the occiput is the denominator and lies closest to the mother's sacrum and even with good contractions does not rotate anteriorly.

personality the unique set of behaviours and attitudes which characterize an individual. They are the result of both inherited traits and environmental influences. The relative dominance of these two causes, nature and nurture, has been controversial for many years.

perspire to sweat.

pertussis (SYNONYM whooping cough) a serious respiratory infection of bacterial origin which can be vaccinated against.

pessary a vaginal insert which can be a mechanical device used to maintain the uterus in an anteverted position or a large tablet-shaped object containing a drug which will be slowly released and absorbed through the vaginal mucus.

PET (pre-eclamptic toxaemia) now called PIH (pregnancy-induced hypertension) – *see* pregnancy-induced hypertension.

petechiae small red spots on the skin. Present on the face after delivery when the baby has had venous congestion. If it is present over the entire body it may suggest infection with rubella, cytomegalovirus or toxoplasmosis.

pethidine hydrochloride (meperidine) an analgesic and anti-spasmodic drug used to treat severe pain, i.e. strong labour. It can cause respiratory depression in the neonate (for which naloxone may be administered) and poor sucking at the breast. Its storage, use and administration are controlled by statute (Misuse of Drugs Regulations 1973) as it is a drug of addiction.

Pethilorfan (Demerol®) a preparation of pethidine and levallorphan used to treat severe pain with less risk of side-effects.

petit mal a mild form of epileptic fit. The person becomes unaware and unresponsive to their surroundings for a short period of time, as opposed to a grand mal attack which is a severe form of epilepsy.

petroleum jelly a by-product of refining crude oil. Used as a barrier or lubricating agent.

Pfannenstiel's incision a surgical cut made across the lower abdomen just above the symphysis pubis. The most frequently used skin incision in caesarean section operations.

PG prostaglandin.

PG² (prostacyclin) hormonally based gel or pessary inserted into the posterior fornix of the vagina to stimulate contractions of the uterus.

PGCE(A) postgraduate certification in education of adults; it is a prerequisite to teaching student midwives.

Ph a tool of measurement used to express the concentration of hydrogen ions in a fluid, also referred to as the acid–alkaline balance. On a 14 point scale, 1 is strongly acid, 7 is neutral and 14 is strongly alkaline. Enzymes, gases and metabolic activity are enhanced by certain acid–alkaline media.

phagocytosis the process by which phagocytes will engulf and kill bacteria or other foreign materials.

phallic referring to the penis or an erect, penis-like shape.

phantom an image or impression; a device for stimulating the interaction of certain tissues with radiation.

phantom pregnancy the impression of being pregnant without evidence.

pharmacokinetics the study of drugs and how they behave in the body and with each other.

Pharmacopoeia a monthly publication listing all available drugs with their uses, side-effects, contraindications and precautions for use.

pharmacy a place for preparing and dispensing drugs.

pharynx the throat – a tube which extends from the base of the skull past the back of the mouth into the oesophagus. It allows the passage of air and food and can change shape during speech.

Phenergan® (promethazine hydrochloride) an antihistamine used in the treatment of allergies and sometimes combined with pethidine in labour to enhance its effect and to treat nausea.

phenobarbital (phenobarbitone) a strong sedative drug used in the management of epilepsy and eclampsia. It should be avoided in early pregnancy.

phenobarbitone *see* phenobarbital.

phenomenology a means of research by which the whole experience is studied. It focuses on describing experiences in order to deepen understanding of them.

phenotype an observable characteristic of an organism which may be physiological, biochemical or behavioural as a result of a combination of inherited traits and environmental factors.

phenylalanine an essential amino acid required for growth and development in infants. It is converted to tyrosine by an enzyme from the liver.

phenylketonuria (PKU) a congenital metabolic disorder characterized by the presence of phenylketones in the urine resulting from the incomplete conversion of phenylalanine to tyrosine. The blood levels will also be elevated and can lead to permanent mental retardation. The condition can be detected before this point by performance of the Guthrie test once feeding has been established for several days. All women should be offered screening for their baby. The 1 in 10 000 babies who suffer from this condition are treated with a phenylalanine-free diet.

phenytoin sodium (Epanutin®) drug used to control and prevent epileptic fits. Where possible it should be avoided in pregnancy.

phimosis tight foreskin which cannot be drawn back over the glans penis. Hygiene is difficult so infections can occur.

phimosis vaginalis a congenital condition in which the vagina is narrow or closed.

phlebitis inflammation of a vein, usually superficial but may be a deep vein in which case there is a risk of thrombosis (clot) developing.

phlebothrombosis a clot of blood within a vein. It is usually in the calf muscle. There is a high risk of the clot becoming detached, travelling in the circulation to the lungs and becoming a pulmonary embolism.

phlebotomist a person who is trained to take blood from a vein.

phlebotomy the process of taking blood from a person.

phlegmasia alba dolens inflammation which causes a white leg as a result of a clot in the femoral vein.

phobia fear or dread which can be so strong that it disables daily functioning. The person may need counselling, behavioural therapy or psychiatric help.

phocomelia a baby born with gross abnormality in development of the long bones. Hands, fingers, feet and toes may be present.

phosphorus a chemical element found in nature. It is essential in the body for using protein, calcium and glucose.

photophobia an intense dislike of light, a symptom of meningitis.

phototherapy treatment using light rays (*see* Figure 104). This accelerates the breakdown of unconjugated bilirubin so that the kidney can excrete it. Bilirubin is a by-product resulting from breakdown of fetal haemoglobin which, until removed from the circulation, binds to fat and colours the skin and sclera of the eye yellow. It is commonly referred to as jaundice.

physician a doctor who specializes in treatment of medical conditions.

physiologic jaundice yellow skin discoloration occurring in 60% of neonates as excess red blood cells are broken down and the liver is not quite mature enough to conjugate them so they can be excreted through the kidney.

physiological breech birth the spontaneous birth of a baby presenting by the breech without interference, medical intervention or attempt at extraction unless a problem occurs.

physiological third stage spontaneous expulsion of the placenta and membranes without intervention. Signs of separation of the placenta from the uterine wall become apparent by lengthening of the umbilical cord, a gush of blood and the uterus rising in the abdomen to be palpable as a small hard mass.

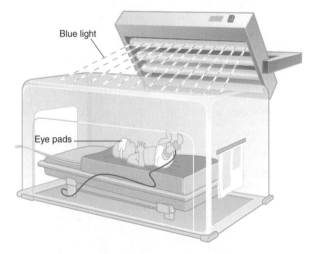

Blue light

Eye pads

■ **Figure 104** Phototherapy

physiology the study of how the body works.

phytomenadione (Konakion®) a preparation of vitamin K given to neonates to prevent haemorrhagic disease of the newborn. It can be given orally or by injection.

pica a craving to eat substances not normally considered fit for food, e.g. clay, chalk.

pie chart a means of representing numerical information on paper in the form of a circle so that percentages of the whole are easily visualized.

Pierre Robin syndrome congenital abnormalities including a small mandible, cleft lip and palate, and other defects of the eyes and ears. Intelligence quotient is usually normal.

piezoelectric effect (*see* Figure 105).

pigment colouring of the skin and hair resulting from the presence of melanin.

piles (haemorrhoids) varicosities protruding from the anus.

Pinard's stethoscope a trumpet-shaped instrument used for listening to the fetal heart sounds through the abdominal wall.

pineal body a cone-shaped structure in the brain whose function is unknown but is thought to be related to sexual arousal.

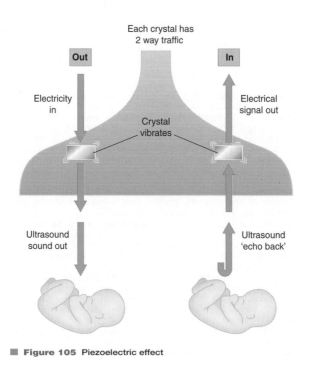

■ **Figure 105** Piezoelectric effect

pinhole pupil very small pupil which may be congenital or the result of drugs.

pinprick test used on the abdomen to test sensation in order to determine the effectiveness of an epidural. A pin and cotton wool are applied to the skin and the women asked to differentiate between them.

pitting oedema small depressions left when fingers are pressed into tissues swollen by the presence of increased intercellular fluid.

pituitary gland pea-sized gland situated at the base of the forebrain behind the bridge of the nose. It secretes hormones which control the other endocrine organs.

PKU *see* phenylketonuria, Guthrie test.

placebo a substance given to a person which has of itself no therapeutic properties but which may relieve symptoms because the person has been told that it will.

placenta the large glandular organ approximately 18 cm in diameter and 2.5 cm thick which grows in the upper segment of the uterus during pregnancy and is attached to the baby by the umbilical cord. It shares circulation with the fetus and its functions are to provide the fetus with the essentials for survival. After delivery of the baby the placenta is squeezed and separates from the wall of the uterus. In *abruptio placentae* the placenta starts to separate partially or completely during pregnancy, thereby reducing the blood supply to the fetus who may die. In *battledore placenta* the cord is attached to the edge rather than centrally located. In *succenturiate placenta* the placenta has an additional lobe situated next to or near the main placenta (*see* Figure 106). The succenturiate

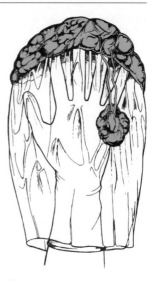

■ **Figure 106** Placenta – succenturiate placenta

lobe may be detached from the main placental tissue and be retained during the third stage of labour, increasing the risk of haemorrhage and infection.

placenta accreta a placenta which grows into the uterine muscle making separation extremely difficult.

placenta bipartita a placenta which appears to have two halves or lobes.

placenta circumvallata a placenta which has a dense white ring on the internal surface caused by a double fold of chorium.

placenta praevia describes a placenta which implants in the lower uterine segment. Its margins may encroach on the cervical os or the placenta may entirely overlie the os. The placenta may separate early in labour as the os starts to dilate

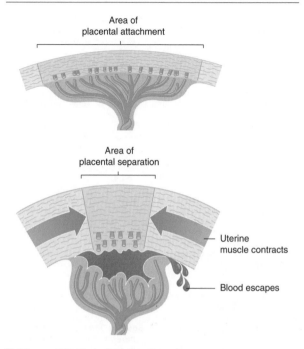

Area of
placental attachment

Area of
placental separation

Uterine
muscle contracts

Blood escapes

■ **Figure 107** Placental separation

causing bleeding and thereby reducing the blood supply to the fetus causing fetal compromise or death.

placental barrier refers to the membranes of the placenta; they permit some substances to enter while excluding others.

placental lactogen a hormone similar to growth hormone which causes growth and development of the breasts during pregnancy.

placental infarct death of an area of the placenta. If this is extensive it will reduce the supply of nutrients and result in fetal compromise including intrauterine growth restriction.

placental insufficiency inability of the placenta to meet fetal demands. Development is compromised in severe cases.

placental membranes the amnion and the chorion which line the uterine cavity.

placental separation the means by which the placenta becomes detached from the uterine wall following the birth of a baby (*see* Figure 107).

placentography radiological means of examining the placenta after injecting it with dye.

placentophagy refers to the eating of the placenta to ingest the hormones. It is believed to elevate the blood levels of oestrogen and progesterone and possibly prevent postnatal depression.

plantar refers to the sole of the foot.

plasma straw-coloured part of the blood made up of water, electrolytes, gases, proteins, glucose, fats and bilirubin. In it are suspended blood cells, erythrocytes, leukocytes and platelets.

plasma expander fluids of high molecular weight given intravenously to raise the blood pressure in situations of shock or haemorrhage.

plasma protein the collective name given to albumin, fibrinogen, prothrombin and gamma globulins, substances which maintain water balance, blood pressure and create osmotic pressure.

plasma volume the amount of plasma in the body. It will be reduced by shock, haemorrhage and dehydration.

plasmin an enzyme which dissolves the fibrin in a thrombus (clot).

PlastiBell™ a plastic device used for circumcision of male babies.

platelets (thrombocytes) cells in the blood which are disc-shaped and are essential to coagulation. They stick to uneven or damaged surfaces causing occlusion through the formation of a clot.

platypelloid word used to describe a pelvis with wide lateral diameters and reduced anterior–posterior diameters. Women with platypelloid pelves rarely have difficulty in labour but the fetal head is unlikely to engage before labour.

plethora excess, usually of red blood cells.

plethoric having the appearance of being saturated with blood.

pleura two membranes, one surrounding the lungs and the other the thorax. The membranes are in very close proximity to each other with only a little fluid between to lubricate them.

pleural cavity the space in the thorax occupied by the lungs and heart.

plexus a place where a number of nerves meet. The *brachial plexus* is the nerves which supply the arm.

pneumococcal meningitis serious infection of the meningeal membranes by pneumococci bacteria.

pneumococcus common term for the bacterial infection-causing organism *Diplococcus pneumoniae*.

pneumonia inflammation of the lung due to infection. May affect all or part of the tissue.

pneumonitis inflammation of the lung, not necessarily due to infection but may be triggered by allergy or pollutants.

podalic internal version of a transverse lie to a longitudinal lie.

poison any substance taken into the body which causes changes in function detrimental to the body's welfare.

polarity term used to describe the harmonious working of the dominant upper uterine segment and the passive lower segment. Uterine contractions in the fundus are strong, and lose strength as they travel towards the lower segment which relaxes and dilates with the cervix as the labour progresses (*see* Figure 108).

poliomyelitis a viral infection of the spinal cord. It is transmitted by the oral–faecal route and may present as nothing more than a common cold. It can, however, cause large muscles of a limb to become paralysed or involve the

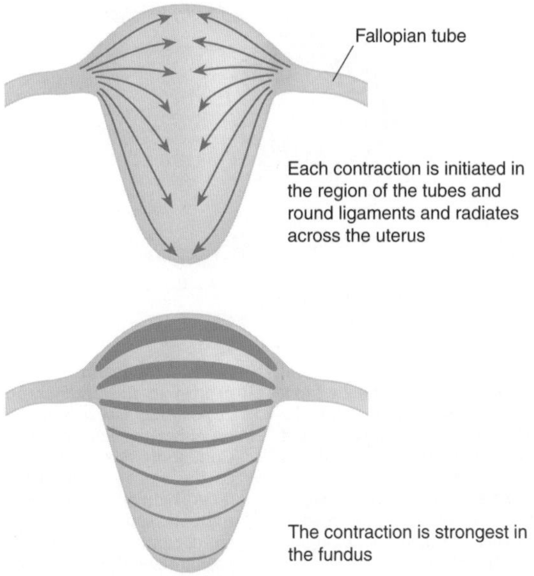

Fallopian tube

Each contraction is initiated in the region of the tubes and round ligaments and radiates across the uterus

The contraction is strongest in the fundus

■ **Figure 108** Polarity

muscles of respiration and the patient frequently dies. It is a notifiable disease. Live attenuated virus is used in preparation of oral vaccines offered to infants at 2, 3 and 4 months of age; the vaccine itself occasionally transmits the disease.

pollutant a substance in the air which when inhaled undermines the body's well-being.

poly- combining form meaning many or much.

polycystic many small cysts or swellings containing fluid or other material.

polycstic kidneys kidneys which are enlarged by many small cysts.

polycystic ovaries ovaries which contain many small cysts. They do not function and the woman will be infertile.

polycythaemia an excess of red blood cells. Newborn babies are usually polycythaemic, the haemoglobin being of the fetal type which is quickly broken down but not so quickly excreted, leading to physiological jaundice.

polydactyly having an extra digit on the hand or the foot.

polyhydramnios having an excess of fluid in the uterine cavity during pregnancy (*see* Figure 109). It may be suggestive of fetal abnormality (e.g. oesophageal atresia).

polymorphic the ability to appear in two or more forms, such as the existence of two or more forms of chromosomes or haemoglobins in a population.

polyneuritis inflammation involving many nerves.

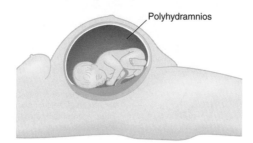

Polyhydramnios

■ **Figure 109** Polyhydramnios

polypus (SYNONYM polyp) a small tumour on a stalk attached to a mucous membrane. May be found on the cervix, containing placental tissue, or resemble a small fibroid.

polyuria passing a lot of urine.

pons that part of the brain lying between the medulla oblongata and the mid-brain.

popliteal space the space at the back of the knee joint.

portal vein the large vein which carries nutritive material from the digestive tract to the liver.

port-wine stain (SYNONYM naevus flammeus) a patch of red/purple discoloration of the skin present at birth.

position usually refers to the attitude of the woman in labour, standing, squatting, forward-leaning, hands and knees, lying prone, supine, recumbent, knee–chest (in cases of cord prolapse to prevent the cord being occluded), left lateral side, lithotomy or Trendelenburg.

position of the fetus the relationship of the presenting part of the fetus to six points on the maternal pelvis. The presenting part, head or breech, has landmarks (denominator: occiput, mentum, sinciput, sacrum) used to describe the fetal aspect nearest to a given point on the pelvis. This landmark may be nearest to the anterior, lateral or posterior aspect of the pelvis on either the left or right side. Commonly six positions are used: right occipitoanterior (ROA), right occipitolateral (ROL), right occipitoposterior (ROP), left occipitoposterior (LOP), left occipitolateral (LOL), and left occipitoanterior (LOA). If the denominator is the sacrum the same positions are used but sacro- (S) is used instead of occipito-. The same applies to the other denominators.

positive end-expiratory pressure (PEEP) the pressure remaining in the airways at the end of an inspiration–expiration cycle during mechanical ventilation.

positive signs of pregnancy audible fetal heart sounds, fetal movements and visualization of the fetus on ultrasound.

possiting regurgitation of a small amount of milk from the stomach of an infant after a feed.

posterior fontanelle the soft fibromembranous point at the back of the infant's head above the occiput where three sutures meet (*see* Figure 110). It may be used to define the baby's position on vaginal examination. It hardens 6 weeks after birth.

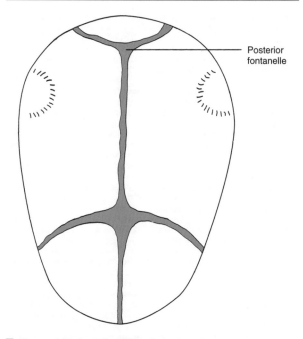

■ **Figure 110** Posterior fontanelle

posterior position the posterior fontanelle of the head lies nearest the mother's spine. The presenting diameter will not be optimal for labour. Backache, slow cervical dilation and descent of the head may be a feature of the labour as the head attempts to rotate to adapt to the shape of the pelvis.

post- combining form meaning after.

postcoital contraception use of hormonal drugs after unprotected intercourse in an attempt to prevent fertilization or implantation.

posterior at the back of.

posthumous after death.

postmature infant a neonate who displays features of dry peeling skin, long fingernails and toenails and skin folds that may crack.

postmenopausal vaginitis inflammation of the vagina associated with degenerative conditions due to hormonal reduction occurring after the cessation of periods.

postmortem (PM; SYNONYM autopsy) examination after death to determine cause of the death.

postnatal after birth.

postnatal depression the negative mood and loss of motivation experienced by 10% of mothers after childbirth. It starts between 10 days and 6 months after birth and can last up to 2 years.

postnatal period the time from birth up to 28 days during which the midwife should attend the mother and child.

postnatal psychosis a serious mental condition in which the woman is unaware of reality and can be a danger to herself or the baby. She may be admitted to a mother and baby psychiatric unit.

postoperative care the care provided after surgery until restoration of full consciousness and functioning state.

postpartum after labour.

postpartum haemorrhage (PPH) severe bleeding from the genital tract up to 6 weeks after labour, of 500 ml of blood or any amount which causes deterioration to the mother's health. May be a threat to the life of the mother so emergency management is required. Primary PPH occurs within 24 hours of birth and is due to relaxation of the myometrium. Secondary PPH occurs after the first 24 hours and up to 6 weeks postpartum and is due to infection or retained products of conception.

postprandial after a meal.

post-traumatic stress disorder a mental response caused by experiencing an acute emotional stress. It happens to people after a natural disaster and may occur in women who have experienced traumatic birth or abusive treatment during their childbirth experience.

postulate a theory; to theorize.

post-term describes a pregnancy which has lasted longer than the medically-defined notion of 'term', usually considered to be between 37 and 42 weeks of pregnancy.

posture the position of the body and the limbs in relation to the trunk.

Potter's syndrome a set of features found in a baby without kidneys. They include poorly developed lungs, compression deformity and unusual facial characteristics. It is not compatible with life.

pouch a small pocket of tissue of membrane.

Poupart's ligament (SYNONYM inguinal ligament) found on the lower abdomen, it stretches from the superior ischial spines to the symphysis pubis.

poverty lacking in the resources and comforts which are expected as basic features of life.

PPH see postpartum haemorrhage.

practitioner a person who has undergone a period of training and has satisfied the relevant professional regulatory body of their competence in the art and science required by that profession of its practitioners.

pragmatic a philosophy which believes that ideas are only valuable in terms of their consequences.

preceptor a person who helps the learning of another without formal classes but by support and discussion.

preceptorship the system by which newly qualified practitioners are supported within the profession until they feel totally confident.

precipitate labour a labour which is very fast, lasting less than 2 hours, and in which the contractions are intense.

preconception the time before embarking on a pregnancy and during which the woman is getting ready to conceive, possibly by adjusting her habits to a healthier way of life.

preconceptual care education and supportive advice provided by a health care worker or lay adviser to a women or couples who are planning to become pregnant.

predisposition a state of being susceptible or inclined to something.

pre-eclampsia (ALSO CALLED PET, pre-eclamptic toxaemia, and PIH, pregnancy-induced hypertension) a syndrome peculiar to pregnancy and characterized by raised blood pressure, generalized oedema and proteinuria. Its cause is unknown but it is associated with high-risk pregnancies in which full fetal development and maternal health are compromised.

Pregaday® medication containing iron and folic acid offered to women thought to be at risk of anaemia in pregnancy.

pregnancy the state lasting 280 days during which the female nourishes in her body a fetus from conception until birth. An *ectopic pregnancy* is one where the conceptus is implanted in the fallopian tube or somewhere outside the uterus.

pregnancy-induced hypertension (PIH) the rise in blood pressure which occurs in some pregnancies. Diastolic blood pressure rises 20 mmHg above the booking pressure or above 90 mmHg. Investigations will be initiated to determine fetal well-being and the condition of the maternal kidneys, liver and coagulation status.

pregnancy test test done on blood or urine to detect a pregnancy. It is based on the detection of human chorionic gonadotrophin (HCG) produced by the trophoblast.

pregnanediol a progesterone-like substance found in the urine of pregnant women.

premature early, the time before full development has been achieved.

premature infant an infant born before 37 completed weeks' gestation.

premature rupture of the membranes the escape of amniotic fluid from around the fetus before the onset of labour.

premedication (premed) medicine, usually a sedative tranquillizer or hypnotic, given before an operation to reduce anxiety and prepare the body. Not usually given before a caesarean section because of the risk of side-effects occurring in the fetus.

premenstrual the time 7–10 days before the start of the regular monthly bleeding which is part of the menstrual cycle.

premenstrual syndrome (PMS) uncomfortable symptoms of weight gain, breast tenderness, volatile mood swings and fatigue which may occur before menstruation.

prenatal before birth.

prenatal diagnosis test performed to confirm or exclude the possibility of a congenital abnormality following a positive screening test.

preoperative the time before an operation.

preoperative care routine procedures which are done before an operation to avoid the complications of anaesthetics; planning of the surgical procedure.

PREP (Post-Registration Education and Practice) a collection of evidence of ongoing education and reflective practice required to be kept by every midwife. It may at any time be requested by the regulatory authorities as part of the requirement of periodic registration.

prepuberty the 2 years before menstruation during which secondary sex characteristics start to appear.

prepuce (SYNONYM foreskin) a loose fold of skin covering the end of the glans penis.

pre-registration midwifery education a midwifery training course of 3 years for women and men wishing to become midwives; in a few areas 18 month programmes are still offered to qualified nurses.

prescription the order by which medicine is issued and given.

presentation the part of the fetus which is lying in the lower segment of the uterus over the cervical os – can be cephalic (head) or breech.

presenting part the part of the fetus which can be palpated in the lower part of the uterus.

pressure force or stress which can be measured and compared to others.

pressure point the area over a bone where the arterial pulse may be felt. May be used for diagnosis and treatement in non-Western healing modalities. Specifically indicated points may be used in acupuncture or acupressure.

presumptive signs indications of a pregnancy, not necessarily beyond question, i.e. amenorrhoea and morning sickness.

preterm before the full 37 weeks of gestation are completed.

preterm labour labour occurring before the 37th completed week of pregnancy. The fetus will be underweight.

prevalence the number of cases of a condition arising at a given time.

preventive measures to take measures so that a disease does not occur.

primary first or most important.

primary health care care based in the community which is offered first in the treatment of a disease. This may include investigation and referral to a hospital based consultant.

primary health care teams small multidisciplinary groups of people who work from health centres and are a person's first communication with midwifery or medical care.

primigravida a woman experiencing her first pregnancy.

primipara a woman who has given birth to a fetus of more than 28 weeks' gestation, live or stillborn.

primiparous having delivered one child.

primitive most basic, rudimentary, no evolution.

primitive groove the dent at the back of the embryonic disk which will become the cephalocaudal axis (head and spine).

primitive reflexes the behaviours with which the baby is born – sucking, breathing, crying, grasping, walking and Moro reflex.

privacy a cultural concept which allows a person to control the number of people around them and prevents intrusive behaviour by one person towards another.

private practice the work of a professional person who is not employed by an institution but is self-employed, may advertise services and make charges.

p.r.n. (LATIN, *pro re nata*) an abbreviation used in prescriptions meaning give as needed.

probability a term used in reporting statistics which measures the likelihood of two or more parameters being related by more than chance.

problem based learning (PBL) students are presented with a problem (trigger) and collectively discover what information they need to resolve the problem. They negotiate which member of their learning set will find which information and feed this back to the group on an agreed date. This process is facilitated by an educationalist. (*See also* evidence based learning (EBL) and inquiry based learning (IBL).)

procaine benzylpenicillin (procaine penicillin) a form of penicillin (antibiotic) given by intramuscular injection which is slow release; used to treat syphilis and gonorrhoea.

procedure a sequential set of actions which together have a single purpose.

process 1. a series of events which will change one thing into another, one state will become another, or a condition will be resolved. 2. part of a bone.

prochlorperazine (Stemetil®) a medicine prescribed to control nausea and vomiting.

procidentia the prolapse of an organ, usually the uterus which comes through the vagina.

procreation the process of conceiving, growing, birthing and nurturing children.

prodromal labour the early stage of labour when contractions occur but are without strength and thus not felt by the woman.

prodrome the first symptoms which may lead to the diagnosis of a disease.

profession a large group of people with similar interests who have organized themselves, documented information and skills, regulated themselves (and by statute) and initiate novices after a course of training. They usually have skills which can be of service to the public and for which the public are willing to pay.

professional a person belonging to a profession who maintains the standards of service and practice adopted by that body.

professional liability the legal obligation of health care professionals to compensate their clients for acts of negligence in their professional practice which cause the clients suffering or damage. This is central to the concept of malpractice.

professional profile documented evidence of the professional person's practice and ongoing training or study.

profile a sketch, summary or diagram of a person or disease.

progeny offspring, children or descendants.

progesterone a hormone produced by the ovaries or placenta which is responsible for the thickening of the endometrium in the uterus, breast changes, water and electrolyte balance and the deposit of fat. It may be given as a medication to treat repeated abortions or for menstrual problems.

progesterone only contraceptive a pill taken at the same time daily which aims to prevent the lining of the endometrium thickening to support implantation of a fertilized ovum. It can be taken by breastfeeding mothers as it does not inhibit milk secretion.

progestogen a natural or synthetic progestational hormone.

prognosis a prediction of the likely future or course of a disease or condition.

Project 2000 a new way of training nurses giving them supernumerary status and a bursary. After a 1-year common foundation course they study their speciality to diploma level and become qualified to provide care to that specific client group.

projectile vomiting strong spasm of the stomach muscles causing the contents to be ejected to a distance of many feet away from the patient. This symptom in a neonate indicates the presence of pyloric stenosis.

prolactin a hormone produced by the anterior lobe of the pituitary gland which is responsible for milk secretion.

prolapse falling of an organ from its usual position through a canal.

prolapse of rectum the protrusion of the rectal mucosal lining through the anus.

prolapse of the umbilical cord the umbilical cord falls through the cervical os in front of the presenting part and may become occluded by it if birth is not expedited or an emergency caesarean section is not performed.

proliferation highly productive, fast multiplication of cells.

proliferation phase refers to the second part of the menstrual cycle when the lining of the uterus is becoming thick and rich with blood.

prolonged labour slow cervical dilation taking more than 24 hours. Occasional risks to the mother include exhaustion, dehydration and ketosis. Risks to the fetus include hypoxia and abnormal moulding which may cause tears to the tentorium of the cerebellum and internal haemorrhage.

prolonged pregnancy pregnancy which lasts more than 42 weeks from the first day of the last normal menstrual period.

promontory that which sticks out. The *sacral promontory* is the part of the sacral vertebrae which protrudes into the pelvic cavity at the brim and reduces the anteroposterior diameter.

prone lying on the front aspect of the body, face downwards.

pronucleus the haploid nucleus of a sex cell.

prophylaxis a treatment given to prevent disease.

propranolol a drug used to lower blood pressure and in some cardiac conditions.

prostacyclin *see* epoprostenol (prostacyclin).

prostaglandin inhibitor an agent which prevents the production of prostaglandin and is usually a non-steroidal anti-inflammatory agent.

prostaglandins (PG) a group of substances first isolated in semen and which have an oxytocic effect, e.g. they cause increased smooth muscle tone and contractions.

prostate gland part of the male reproductive system located at the neck of the bladder which produces seminal fluid in which sperm may be transported and can swim.

Prostin E® a drug made to resemble and have the same action as prostaglandins. Used in the treatment of abortions and induction of labour by increasing the sensitivity of the myometrium to oxytocin.

protamine sulphate (Prosulf®) a drug to counteract the effects of heparin.

protein the part of the diet required for growth and repair of tissue. Contains the elements hydrogen, oxygen, nitrogen and carbon. It is digested in the stomach and absorbed in the form of amino acids, the most common being albumin (responsible for normal distribution of water throughout the body and the maintenance of the blood pressure).

proteinuria an abnormal condition where protein is excreted in the urine.

Proteus a bacterium found normally in the faeces but if transported to other parts of the body by contamination can cause urinary tract infections, pyelonephritis, wound infections and diarrhoea.

prothrombin a protein found in the plasma of the blood which in certain conditions will become thrombin in the presence of calcium and form part of a blood clot.

protocol a written plan which describes best treatment for a certain condition.

proximal next to, closest to.

pruritus itching sensation on the skin which causes the person to scratch.

pseudo- combining form meaning false.

pseudocyesis (false pregnancy) the woman feels she is pregnant and may develop symptoms of amenorrhoea and enlarged abdomen but there is no fetus in the uterus.

pseudohermaphroditism an individual with congenitally malformed genitalia, expressing both male and female characteristics.

pseudomenstruation bleeding which resembles a period but without changes in the lining of the uterus.

psch-, psycho- prefix meaning relating to the mind.

psychiatry a specialized branch of medicine which looks at disease processes of the mental, emotional or behavioural functions of the individual.

psychomotor relating to motor activities, movements initiated at will.

psychomotor development the ongoing changes and refinement in mental and muscular harmony or cooperation. Usually refers to the progressive muscular control acquired at different ages.

psychologist a professional who studies the structure of the brain and the functions of the mind.

psychoprophylactic preparation for childbirth education of parents concerning the processes of birth and how to cope with/remain in control of them.

psychoprophylaxis a system for coping with pain in labour based on education in the Lamaze method of relaxation.

psychosexual relating to the mental and emotional aspects of sexuality.

psychosis severe mental illness characterized by delusions, hallucinations and illusions and loss of contact with reality. Postpartum, some women develop puerperal or postnatal psychosis.

psychosocial development progressive changes in a child's ability to interact with other people and develop relationships of trust and respect.

ptyalin the enzyme in saliva which starts the process of starch digestion in the mouth.

puberty the transition in physical, mental and emotional functioning of the body which happens between about 10 and 18 years of age. The child emerges into adulthood.

pubescent uterus the body and cervix of the uterus are the same size and length in the adult as in the child.

pubic region the lowest part of the abdomen between the right and left inguinal regions.

pubic symphysis (SYNONYM symphysis pubis) the cartilaginous structure in the anterior mid-line of the pelvis. It may soften in pregnancy and the bones part causing symphysis pubis dysfunction.

pubiotomy the opening of the pubic bone in order to increase the pelvic diameters to let the fetus pass through the birth canal.

pubis the bone at the front of the pelvis.

public health intervention in the environment and clinical practice which will affect the health of the population or community.

pubococcygeus that part of the pelvic floor muscle (levator ani) which stretches from the pubis to the coccyx.

pudendal refers to the external genital organs.

pudendal block anaesthetic injected into the region of the pudendal nerve before the application of forceps to anaesthetize the lower genital tract.

pudendum the external genitalia.

puerperal referring to the period of time after childbirth.

puerperal fever elevation of the temperature and other signs of severe infection following childbirth.

puerperal psychosis a severe mental illness which can follow childbirth.

puerperal pyrexia a rise in the body temperature after childbirth.

puerperal sepsis infection, usually in the genital tract, after childbirth.

puerperium the period of time lasting 6–8 weeks after childbirth during which the body begins to return to its non-pregnancy state and breastfeeding is established.

pulmonary referring to the lungs.

pulmonary circulation the flow of blood through the lungs so that oxygen can be taken up and pumped to the rest of the body and carbon dioxide given off.

pulmonary embolism a clot of blood which has travelled from another part of the body (the legs) and has become wedged in the small capillaries of the lungs, preventing flow and oxygenation of blood. It is accompanied by chest pain, cyanosis and tachypnoea. It can be life-threatening.

pulmonary surfactant a chemical found in the lung which maintains elasticity and inhibits collapse of the alveoli thereby facilitating gaseous exchange.

pulsation a throbbing or beating of an artery as blood passes through; it is rhythmic and in time with the beating of the heart.

pulse the rhythmic wave felt in an artery as the heart contracts forcing blood along it.

pulse rate the number of times per minute the heart pumps; the speed of the cardiac cycle.

pump apparatus used to move fluids from one place to another.

puncture making a hole in something by piercing it with a sharp instrument. In a *lumbar puncture* a hole is made in the meninges in the lumbar region of the spine in order to obtain cerebrospinal fluid for diagnostic or therapeutic purposes.

PUO (pyrexia of unknown origin) a body temperature above normal in response to something unknown.

purchaser people, usually GPs, who pay money for treatments to be administered to their patients by the provider (the hospital).

purgative a medicine which causes the bowels to be evacuated or emptied.

purpura haemorrhagica purple spots or patches appearing on the skin or mucous membrane caused by bleeding of small capillaries beneath.

pus an exudate of yellow/white thick fluid which contains leukocytes, dead bacteria and skin cells. Produced in response to the body's resistance to an infection.

pustule small round patches on the skin with yellow tops indicating that pus is contained within.

p.v. (per vaginam) refers to medicine administered or examinations conducted by passing through the vagina.

pyaemia pus in the blood, a by-product of bacterial invasion.

pyelitis infection in the renal pelvis of the kidney.

pyelonephrosis any disease of the kidney.

pyloric stenosis narrowing of that part of the gut that allows nutrients out of the stomach into the intestines for further digestion. Projectile vomiting and weight loss are the diagnostic features.

pylorus the opening between the stomach and the duodenum.

pyo- combining form meaning pus.

pyocolpos accumulation of pus in the vagina.

pyogen organisms/bacteria which produce pus.

pyogenic pus forming.

pyometra accumulation of pus in the uterus.

pyosalpinx pus in the fallopian tubes.

pyretic referring to the presence of a fever or abnormally raised body temperature.

pyrexia fever, elevation in body temperature above normal (37°C) in order to resist infection.

pyridoxine a preparation of vitamin B_6 given to treat anaemia.

pyuria pus in the urine, indicating the presence of infection in the urinary tract. The urine is cloudy.

Qq

QRS complex a series of letters denoting the parts of a cardiac muscular contraction so they can be recorded and analysed on paper (*see* Figure 111).

quadrant a quarter of a circle or a part of the body which can be divided by four; the abdomen or the buttock.

quadruplets four babies developing within the uterus or born in a single pregnancy.

qualified a person who has received a recognized training and successfully completed the criteria for entering into employment requiring skills acquired during the training.

qualitative research a means of gathering and analysing information about life experiences and their meaning. It is done to acquire information of a conceptual nature or about aspects of the human condition which vary from one individual to another.

quality assessment measures a system for evaluating patterns and programmes of clinical, administrative and consumer care.

quality assurance a pledge or assurance given to the public by a group (service provider) that they will work towards certain standards of care which have been agreed by a multidisciplinary group. Once the standards have been agreed, progress towards attainment of those standards is monitored and evaluated to obtain further information about other standards required. In this way all clients should receive the best available care or product.

quantitative research a means of research by which data are collected in numerical form; variables can be compared and interventions measured for effectiveness.

quantitative ultrasound an ultrasound technique for measuring bone density in women at risk of osteoporosis.

quarantine a period of time during which a person or animal thought to have been in contact with an infectious disease is isolated from contact with others. If after the expected time the person/animal has not developed the infection, freedom to be in contact with others is restored.

'quickening' the moment in the pregnancy when the mother first feels the fetus move. It happens around 19 weeks for a primigravida and around 16 weeks for a multigravida.

quiet alertness the hour after a baby is born and several hours a day during which the newborn is calm and attentive, looks around and gets to know the adults around her/him and her/his environment.

quintuplets five babies developing within the uterus or born in a single pregnancy.

quotient a number obtained by division. *Intelligence quotient* is a number used to indicate intellectual capacity. The person is given a test. The score is multiplied by 100 and divided by the person's age and the results compared with others of the same age.

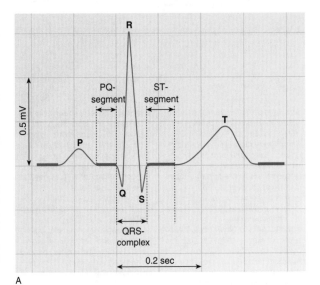

A

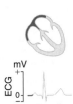

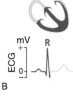

B

■ **Figure 111** QRS complex of the adult heart

Rr

race a group of individuals with genetic and other characteristics in common.

racemose clustered; describes glands arranged around a central duct or orifice.

rachischisis a congenital fusion of one or more vertebrae.

rachitic dwarf a small person whose growth was retarded by the disease rickets.

rachitic pelvis structural deformity of the pelvis caused by rickets in childhood.

radial referring to the radius bone in the lower arm.

radial artery the artery which passes down the arm and can be felt pulsating as it passes over the radius just above the wrist.

radial nerve large nerve supplying the arm and forearm.

radial nerve palsy damage to the nerve resulting in weakness and sensory loss which may be permanent or temporary following shoulder dystocia.

radiant describes an object which emits rays (of heat, light or electricity) or is the centre of rays which spread outwards.

radiate to diverge or spread out from a common point.

radiation the use of radioactive substances in diagnosis or treatment of disease.

radical dealing with the root or cause of a disease.

radical mastectomy surgical removal of the breast and extensive excision including lymph nodes, pectoral muscles and axillary lymph nodes to which cancerous cells may have spread.

radical midwife a midwife who believes in returning to the roots of being with women, enabling informed choice and practising autonomously; using Western medicine only when specifically indicated rather than on a routine basis.

radioactive a substance, usually metal, which emits electromagnetic vibrations.

radiographer a person trained to take and interpret X-rays of the bones and other parts of the body.

radiography examination by X-ray to detect or diagnose a condition. Not recommended in pregnancy without good clinical indications.

radioimmunoassay a means by which antibodies, antigens, hormones and drugs can be detected and measured.

radio-opaque something which stops the passage of X-rays and reflects them back so that an image can be created.

radiotelemetry a method of collecting information using a sensor and transmitting information to a base where it can be interpreted and recorded. Fetal heart monitoring can be recorded by this method.

radius one of the bones (with the ulna) in the forearm.

Ramstedt's operation surgery performed in cases of pyloric stenosis to increase the size of the sphincter muscle which is causing obstruction.

ramus the upper and lower arm-like parts of a bone as in the pubic bone.

random blood sugar test checking of blood sugar level without prior preparation or warning. (*Compare* glucose tolerance test.)

random sampling a system in which research participants have equal chance of being selected for a particular group.

randomization the process by which individuals, e.g. experimental or control subjects, are allocated to one of two groups, without a pattern or predictor of the group to which the subject will be assigned.

randomized controlled trial (RCT) a research method in which one group receives standard care and treatment and another group receives some form of intervention. Which participant is allocated to which group is decided completely by chance in an attempt to reduce bias.

ranitidine drug used in the treatment of duodenal and gastric ulcers. It may be offered to women in labour to reduce acidity of gastric secretion; controversy exists over whether this is indicated nowadays.

rape sexual intercourse by force. The non-consenting party may be physically or psychologically injured by the assault. The term *medical rape* describes abuse arising from the application of medical procedures upon women and babies by force.

rapport a sense of understanding, harmony and respect between two people.

rash raised red area of skin which can cause irritation. *Heat rash* appears in hot steamy conditions. It is also called prickle heat. *Nappy rash* appears over the nappy area and can be caused by irritation of strong urine (ammonia). It is more common where there is poor hygiene, and during colds, teething and earache.

raspberry leaf tea a herbal infusion often used in the latter part of pregnancy and thought to increase uterine muscle tone.

rate a measurement, e.g. of time, speed, velocity, used for the purpose of comparison. *Basal metabolic rate* is a unit of measurement used to indicate the body's requirements for oxygen when at rest. One person's rate can be compared with others and the result will be expressed in relationship to them. The *birth rate* is the number of births in a specific population over a period of time, usually expressed per year per 1000 of the population.

ratio a means of describing the quantity of one substance in relation to another. With the *lecithin–sphingomyelin ratio*, the relationship of these two substances to each other as found in the amniotic fluid is used to indicate fetal lung maturity.

rationale a system of reasoning or a statement of the reasons used in explaining actions or data.

reaction a response occurring secondary to a treatment or stimulus.

Read method a method of preparation for childbirth initially prepared by Dr Grantley Dick Read. It is based on the relaxation, information and pain triangle. Women are prepared for birth by being educated so that through understanding their fear may be reduced as fear is known to make pain worse. Relaxation improves the ability to cope with pain and gentle exercise promotes relaxation and fitness.

reagent a substance which causes a reaction. A substance which in the presence of another to which it is sensitive alters its characteristics thereby indicating the presence of the other substance.

real-time scanner moving images created by ultrasound scanning.

reasonable care the degree of skill and knowledge expected of a qualified person.

recession drawing away from a normal position or turning backwards. *Sternal recession* is a sinking in of the breast bone with each inhalation seen in babies with respiratory distress syndrome.

recessive the opposite to dominant; a characteristic which will only be expressed as a genetic feature if a similar gene is present in both parents.

recipient the one who receives or accepts something given by another.

recommended daily allowance (RDA) the quantity of various nutrients in daily food intake considered by the Food and Nutrition Board of the National Research Council to be necessary for optimal health.

record permanent written communication which can be a document of care.

recovery return to normality or state of consciousness after an anaesthetic.

recreational drug a chemical substance not prescribed and taken for the pleasure it induces rather than for clinical indications.

rectal referring to the rectum, the lowest part of the alimentary canal closed by the anal sphincter. Drugs and infusions may be given and are well absorbed via this route.

rectal atresia the rectal canal ends in a blind loop and is not connected to the anal or distal end of the rectum (*see* Figure 112).

rectal reflex the normal ejection response to the presence

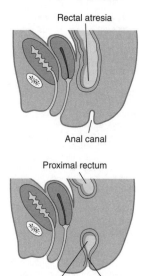

■ **Figure 112** Rectal atresia

of an accumulation of faeces in the rectum. In babies this can be elicited within 20 minutes of a meal.

rectal temperature taken occasionally in the neonate; should be used with extreme caution as it carries risks of perforation. A special thermometer is required and the measurement is 0.4°C higher than the oral temperature.

rectocele a weakness in the muscle wall separating the rectum and vagina which allows the rectum and contents to bulge into the vagina. Surgical colporrhaphy may be performed to correct the defect.

rectovaginal refers to the rectum and vagina and the area where they are in closest proximity. In a rectovaginal fistula a hole appears between the rectum and vagina allowing faecal matter to leak out of the rectum into the vagina and out of the body in an uncontrolled manner.

rectovesical refers to the rectum and bladder.

rectum the lower 15 cm of the large intestine, it collects and contains faeces until it is convenient to evacuate.

rectus abdominis a pair of muscles on the anterior abdominal wall stretching from the ribs to the symphysis pubis. They may divide spontaneously during pregnancy and after delivery they can be palpated up to 4 cm apart. They usually close up within 6 months especially with exercise, but occasionally surgical repair may be required.

recumbent lying down.

red blood cell count the number of erythrocytes in a specimen of blood – should be between 4.6 and 6.2 million/mm^3.

reduce 1. to make smaller. 2. to lower the measured volume or weight of something. 3. restore to the original position, as in fractured bone.

referral a process by which a client or family is introduced to additional or more specialized health care.

reflection 1. a communication technique in which the listener picks up an unexpressed feeling or idea in the client's tone of voice and repeats it back asking for clarification. 2. a method by which practitioners use a model or reflective cycle and apply it to a practice incident with a view to increasing learning or self-awareness.

reflex a backward or return flow of energy.

reflex action an involuntary movement which happens in response to a stimulus, e.g. light shone into the eye causes the pupil to contract.

reflexology a method of treating certain disorders in parts of the body by massaging the soles of the feet.

reflux abnormal backward flow or movement of a fluid.

regional anaesthesia an injection of drugs into a part of the body to prevent sensation being experienced in that area.

register a list on which participants or people with features in common are recorded, e.g. the *disability register*. The *birth register* is the list of names and details of all babies which is given to the registrar of births, marriages and deaths.

Register of Midwives names of all qualified midwives who are deemed fit to practise midwifery.

Registered General Nurse (RGN) a person who has received instruction and successfully completed a course of study in the art and science of caring for people unable to maintain for themselves their optimal state of health.

Registered Midwife (RM) a person who has successfully completed a course of study on the care of women and their families during pregnancy and childbirth and whose name has been entered onto part 10 of the Register of Midwives.

registrar a doctor who has specialized in a particular field of medicine over several years.

registrar of births, marriages and deaths the person in the civic council offices who holds a records of the births, deaths and marriages which have occurred in a designated geographical area. The Office of Population, Censuses and Surveys (OPCS) oversees the work, collects data and conducts demographical surveys.

regurgitation backward flow, maybe against gravity, of a fluid. In pregnancy regurgitation of the gastric juices through a weakened cardiac sphincter causes heartburn.

rehydration the replacement of fluids. Women in labour lose fluid due to high energy expenditure and should be offered fluids regularly in order to prevent the need to be rehydrated by intravenous means.

relaxant a drug which causes relaxation of muscles given during surgery or administered to control muscle spasm.

relaxation referring to a state of being at rest and applicable to the whole body or to individual muscles. Some antenatal classes are designed to help teach relaxation techniques.

relaxin a hormone thought to cause general softening of tissues including cartilage. In pregnancy softening of the symphysis pubis may enable increased diameters of the pelvis.

releasing factor a trigger substance released from the hypothalamus which causes the pituitary to release hormones.

reliability the extent to which a test produces the same results with different researchers, observers and at different times.

REM (rapid eye movement) referring to a type of eye activity observed during sleep.

renal referring to the kidneys.

renal failure the kidney fails to function allowing toxins to remain in the blood where they will act like a poison. It is likely to occur following severe haemorrhage, eclampsia or infection.

renal threshold the point at which the kidney will function correctly. The threshold may be lower in pregnancy allowing substances to stay in the urine when they would normally have been reabsorbed, e.g. glucose.

renin an enzyme made, stored and secreted by the kidney. It is responsible for maintaining the blood pressure.

rennin an enzyme found in the stomach which causes milk to curdle and become insoluble.

repercussion ballottement, rebound of an object through a fluid.

reproduction the process by which two of a species create and nurture a future member of the same species.

reproductive organs the parts of the body involved in reproduction: ovaries, fallopian tubes, uterus, vagina, vulva and breasts in females; penis, testes, scrotum, prostate gland and connecting tubules in males.

research the search for new knowledge.

research instrument a testing device for measuring a given idea, usually a questionnaire, interview, or guidelines for observation.

resect removal of body tissue by surgery.

residual urine urine remaining in the bladder after micturition. More than 100 ml residual urine can indicate dysfunction.

resilience the ability of the body to return to its previous form after being stretched, as in childbirth.

resistance a force exerted against another force, usually referring to the body's ability to overcome bacterial or other infection.

resistant capacity of a microbe not to be affected by an antibiotic drug.

resource management a system initiated in 1986 by government aimed at increasing functional efficiency and effectiveness by devolving management to local groups. The local managers draw up business plans, are responsible and accountable for allocation of resources and are more responsive to local demands, needs and changes.

respiration breathing; the taking in of oxygen and excretion of carbon dioxide from the blood so that oxygen can be passed around the body to enable metabolism. *Artificial respiration* is a mechanical process of gaseous exchange performed when a person is unable to breathe for themselves. The lungs are inflated mechanically by a ventilator. The machine mixes gases, and monitors input and output.

respiration rate the adult average is 20 breaths per minute, while neonates vary between 40 and 60 breaths per minute.

respiratory alkalosis decreased excretion of carbon dioxide causing accumulation in the blood and altering the pH value.

respiratory arrest cessation of breathing; may be due to drugs, allergy or obstruction of the airway.

respiratory centre the area of the brain which controls the rate and depth of breathing.

respiratory distress syndrome (RDS) a condition seen in preterm infants caused by lack of surfactant. Lung expansion cannot be maintained, and oxygen and CO_2 exchange is impaired. The baby becomes exhausted by the efforts of breathing and there is characteristic flaring of the nares, expiratory grant, sternal and intercostal recession.

respiratory tract the interconnecting structures of nose, bronchus, bronchioles, trachea, pharynx and lungs by means of which air enters the body ready for gaseous exchange.

respiratory tract infection any infection of the upper respiratory tract, e.g. sinusitis, laryngitis, tonsillitis, or the lower respiratory tract, e.g. bronchitis, pneumonia.

restitution returning to the correct place. The fetal head immediately after delivery rotates to restore alignment with the shoulders (*see* Figure 113).

resuscitation restoration from a state of collapse. *Neonatal resuscitation* is necessary for infants who fail to breathe spontaneously at birth.

retained placenta describes the situation where the placenta has not been delivered within what is deemed a locally appropriate time after the delivery of the baby. It may need to be removed manually (*see* Figure 114).

retardation delay. *Fetal growth retardation* is when the fetus fails to gain weight. *Mental retardation* is when the brain fails to mature or is permanently damaged. The person will have a low IQ and function at a lower level than chronologically appropriate.

retching attempting to be sick.

retention holding on to, holding back. In *urinary retention* the bladder fails to evacuate urine.

reticuloendothelial system a network of cells found in the connective tissue, lungs, liver, spleen, and bone marrow. They are concerned with the formation and destruction of red blood cells (erythrocyctes), storage of fats, storage of iron, inflammation and immunity. Some cells move in the blood and can ingest foreign materials.

retina the inner lining of the eye which receives light images and sends them to the brain for interpretation.

retinal detachment the retina comes away from the choroids. Further detachment may occur if women with this condition

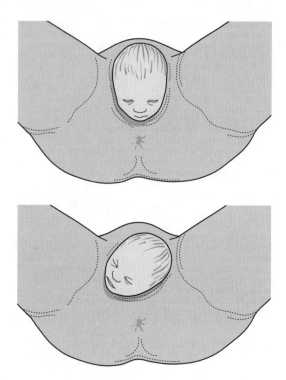

■ **Figure 113** Restitution

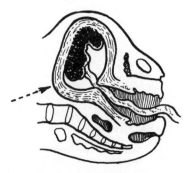

■ **Figure 114** Retained placenta after Syntometrine® injection

push vigorously during the second stage of labour. They may choose assisted delivery or prefer to adopt upright positions which enable the baby to be born without vigorous pushing.

retinopathy refers to damage to the retina.

retinopathy of prematurity iatrogenic retinal opacity and occlusion occurring secondary to oxygen therapy which has been given to the premature newborn.

retracted nipple a nipple which is drawn inwards by fibrotic bands of tissue beneath the skin and does not protrude easily even when stimulated.

retraction pulling back. A state of permanent shortening of uterine muscle fibres occurring during contraction. Following relaxation some of the shortening is retained. The next contraction requires less effort to achieve the same traction (*see* Figure 115) achieving a state of progressive dilatation.

retractor a surgical instrument used to pull back another organ from the field of operation.

retro- combining form meaning behind or at the back.

retrograde moving backwards.

retrograde menstruation the backflow of the menstrual discharge through the uterus, fallopian tubes and into the abdominal cavity.

retroplacental behind the placenta.

retroplacental clot a collection of blood behind the placenta.

retroversion bending backwards.

retroversion of the uterus refers to the whole uterus being bent or tilted backwards instead of forwards (*see* Figure 116).

retroverted gravid uterus when a retroverted uterus containing a pregnancy becomes trapped in the pelvis, its passage being obstructed by the sacral promontory.

retrovirus a group of RNA viruses including the ones causing AIDS and leukaemia. These viruses replicate by inserting DNA copy of their genome into a healthy host cell.

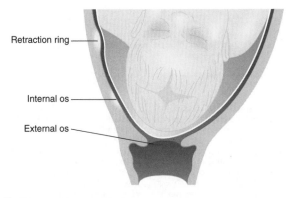

Retraction ring

Internal os

External os

■ **Figure 115** Retraction ring

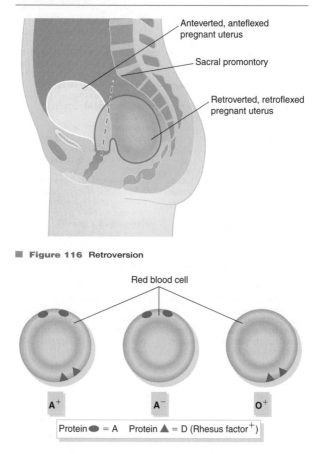

Figure 116 Retroversion

Figure 117 Rhesus factor

rhesus factor (Rh) an antigen which may be present or absent on the red cells causing the blood group to be termed rhesus negative or rhesus positive (*see* Figure 117 and Appendix).

rhesus immune globulin the immune globulin which is offered to rhesus negative mothers after abortion or birth unless the infant is also rhesus negative. It can prevent the mother developing antibodies to the Rh positive factor which may pass into her circulation during placental separation. The immunoglobulin coats the fetal blood cells so that the mother's body does not recognize them as foreign proteins.

rhesus incompatibility the mismatch between two groups of blood cells – mother and fetus or donor to recipient's blood. The Rh factor is present in the blood of one but not the other so agglutination (sticking together of the cells) can occur if fetal blood escapes into the maternal circulation.

rhythm a constantly repeating sequence of events.

rhythm method of family planning a method of avoiding pregnancy based on avoiding intercourse during the ovulatory phase of the menstrual cycle. It is dependent on a predictable cycle, and a record of past cycles. This method may also be combined with observation of the basal body temperature and the texture of the vaginal secretions in order to establish the 'safe' period for sexual intercourse.

ribonucleic acid (RNA) the cytoplasmic acid found in cells which translate the DNA information into action.

rickets deformity of the bones caused by dietary lack of vitamin D in the formative years.

right occipitoanterior (ROA) refers to the position of the fetal skull in relation to the maternal pelvis. The back of the head, the occiput, is positioned to the front and right side of the maternal pelvis.

right occipitolateral (ROL) the fetal occiput in utero is to the right side of the maternal pelvis.

right occipitoposterior (ROP) the occiput is on the right side and to the back of the maternal pelvis.

right sacroanterior (RSA) refers to the position of the fetus when the breech is presenting. The sacrum (the bony eminence above the buttocks) is to the front right side of the mother's pelvis.

right sacrolateral (RSL) when the breech is presenting and the sacrum is on the right and to the side of the mother's pelvis.

right sacroposterior (RSP) the sacrum is on the right side and the back of the mother's pelvis.

right-to-left shunt an abnormal communication/hole between the atria which enables passage of blood from one side to the other.

rigor an attack of shivering and shaking seen in response to a rise in the body temperature.

risk factor a factor in the health or history of an individual which may make her more susceptible to a specific complication occurring. Risk factors in pregnancy include certain medical and previous obstetric conditions. Many of the risk factors cited to women and used to guide practice are not well researched and/or underpinned by sound evidence, therefore risk scoring may not be an appropriate form of care.

risk management a structure designed to identify and eliminate risks ensuring optimal care and preventing medical and legal problems. The structure includes standards of care and clinical guidelines based on research, case note reviews, case conferences and staff training sessions.

Ritgen manoeuvre a technique sometimes used during the second stage of labour whereby upward pressure is applied to the fetal head from the coccygeal region to extend it during actual delivery (*see* Figure 118). Those who practise this manoeuvre tend to do so because they feel it will reduce the incidence of perineal tears.

ritodrine hydrochloride a drug used to prevent uterine activity and so prevent preterm labour.

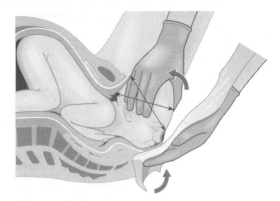

■ **Figure 118** Ritgen manoeuvre

Ritter's disease a severe form of pemphigus neonatorum. A staphylococcal skin infection.

role an exhibited pattern of behaviour enacted to fulfil a given expectation.

role conflict the presence of contradictory elements within one's expected behaviour.

role model a person whose action inspires another to similar behaviour.

rooming-in a system in which the baby remains at the mother's bedside throughout its stay in hospital.

rooting reflex the innate ability of the neonate to search for and find the nipple.

roseola a pink/rose-coloured rash.

rotation turning round. Refers to the ability of the fetal head when deep in the pelvis to be deflected by the pelvic floor muscles so that it turns round to accommodate itself to the shape of the outlet.

rotavirus a wheel-shaped virus that causes diarrhoea in infants.

roughage the indigestible parts of the diet which pass through the intestines encouraging peristalsis.

round ligament a sheet of tissue extending from the cornea of the uterus to the vulva (*see* Figure 119).

Royal College of General Practitioners (RCGP) an organization aiming to support and represent the interests of family doctors. It is similar to the Royal College of Midwives.

Royal College of Midwives (RCM) a professional organization aiming to support the work of midwives. It is funded by the members, its officers are elected by members, and it is concerned with terms of employment, complaints, training, educational conferences, lobbying of parliament and initiating guidelines for good practice. It has an extensive library service.

Royal College of Nursing (RCN) a professional organization for nurses similar to the Royal College of Midwives.

rubella (SYNONYM German measles) a viral infection with symptoms of the common cold

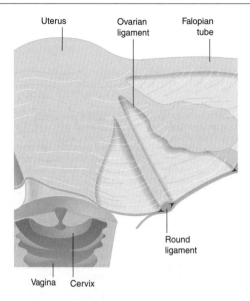

Uterus Ovarian ligament Falopian tube

Round ligament

Vagina Cervix

■ **Figure 119** Round ligament

and macular rash. If it occurs in the first trimester of pregnancy it can cause congenital anomaly of the heart, eye or ear or even stillbirth. It can be vaccinated against at 18 months or 13 years of age.

Rubin's test an examination performed to test the patency of the fallopian tubes. Carbon dioxide is introduced under pressure. If the pressure falls the tubes are patent as the gas has escaped into the abdominal cavity.

rugae (SINGULAR ruga) the folds or creases found in the stomach and in the vaginal wall which allow it to stretch.

Rules for Midwives rules laid down by the Nursing and Midwifery Council. Practitioners must follow them to enjoy the confidence and safeguard the interests of the public. Failure to follow the Midwives Rules and

Code of Practice can lead to investigations and disciplinary action.

rupture tearing or bursting of a tube, membrane or organ such that the contents escape. For example, *rupture of membranes* in labour or *rupture of the uterus* in obstructed labour.

rupture of the uterus the muscle fibres of the uterus divide with loss of integrity of the cavity, displacement and likely death of the fetus, and excessive bleeding and shock in the mother.

ruptured hymen the fragmented membranous tags found in the vagina indicative of penetrative intercourse.

Ryle's tube thin opaque tube which is flexible enough to be passed via the nose into a baby's stomach to administer feeds or aspirate contents.

Ss

Sabin vaccine three live but weakened polio viruses which are given orally in an attempt to enable the body to develop its own immunity to polio.

sac pouch or pocket-like cavity.

sacculation of the uterus a term applied to the incarcerated gravid uterus. The rise of the uterus into the abdominal cavity is obstructed by the sacral promontory. Only the anterior aspect of the uterus will grow with stretching of the urethra and causing retention of urine.

sacral, sacro- referring to the sacrum.

sacral promontory the anterior aspect of the first sacral vertebra which protrudes into the pelvic inlet and is a featured landmark.

sacral vertebrae the five bones of the spinal column which fuse together to form the sacrum and posterior aspect of the pelvis. They have a convex anterior surface.

sacrococcygeal refers to the sacrum and the coccyx.

sacrocotyloid referring to the sacrum and the acetabulum. The distance is occasionally measured and should be 9.5 cm otherwise a contracted pelvis may be suspected.

sacroiliac refers to the sacrum and the ilium.

sacroiliac joint the fixed joint between the ilium and the sacrum which might be slightly movable in pregnancy.

sacrum large wedge-shaped bone composed of five fused vertebrae situated at the lower end of the spinal column and forming the back wall of the pelvic girdle.

Safe Motherhood Initiative an ambitious programme launched by the World Health Organization in 1987 aimed at improving the health of women before pregnancy so that morbidity and mortality can be reduced. In underdeveloped countries, birth attendants are trained to monitor pregnancies and refer to a midwife if abnormality occurs.

safe sex the practice of using condoms during sexual intercourse to prevent the exchange of bodily fluids thereby preventing the possible transmission of diseases including the HIV virus.

Saf-T-Coil an intrauterine contraceptive device.

sagittal an imaginary line extending from the front to the back of the body and bisecting a region, referred to as a sagittal section. The *sagittal suture* is a suture separating the parietal bones.

sagittal fontanelle a soft area on the sagittal suture posterior to the bregma. It may be found in some neonates and babies with Down's syndrome.

salbutamol (Ventolin®) a drug used to make smooth muscle relax. Primarily administered in asthmatics but can also be used in preterm labour or to treat the tonic contractions caused by the use of Syntocinon®.

salicylate a salt found in preparations such as aspirin used as an antipyretic, anti-inflammatory and analgesic. It works by inhibiting prostaglandin manufacture which is responsible for inflammation.

saline a solution containing water and 0.9% salt.

saliva the secretions of the mouth which moisten food and start the process of carbohydrate digestion.

Salmonella bacteria responsible for causing gastroenteritis. The causative organism in several outbreaks of food poisoning with associated fatalities.

salpingectomy removal of the fallopian tube.

salpingitis inflammation of the fallopian tube.

salpingogram procedure whereby a radio contrast medium is introduced via the cervix, pumped into the uterus and X-rays are taken as it passes through the fallopian tubes into the abdomen. It is done to establish patency of the tube.

salpingography X-ray images of the fallopian tubes produced after injection of radio-opaque contrast medium.

salpingo-oophorectomy removal of the fallopian tube and ovary.

salpingotomy cutting into or opening up of the fallopian tube.

salpinx a tube, usually the fallopian tube.

sample a group in the population selected as representative of the entire population. Research will be conducted with the cooperation of the group and results will be generalized to the population.

sanguine abundant blood in the circulation giving a ruddy complexion and an attitude of vitality and confidence.

sanitary napkin (SYNONYM sanitary towel) a pad used to absorb menstrual flow. May be disposable or washable/recyclable.

sanitation the maintenance of a healthy, disease-free environment.

scabies skin infestation with the human itch mite. It is highly contagious. The itch mite burrows just below the skin and can cause a reaction.

scalp the skin over the top of the head out of which the hair grows.

scalpel a very fine, sharp knife used for making surgical incisions (cutting).

scan an examination of a part of the body using computer generated images to determine abnormal conditions. In *ultrasound scanning* (USS) sound waves are used to generate images of structures within the body.

scapula the flat triangular bone found behind the shoulder.

scarlet fever contagious disease of childhood caused by haemolytic Streptococcus A. Typical presentation is a red rash, fever, sore throat, headache and vomiting.

Schedule of Drugs a means of categorizing drugs according to their potential for abuse. There are five groups – Schedules I–V. Schedule I drugs are not available legally as they have a high risk of abuse. Schedule V are available and considered at low risk of abuse.

schizophrenia a psychotic disease in which the person has periods of normality interspersed with varying periods and degrees of hallucinations and delusions.

school health service the provision of health surveillance made by the local education authority whereby nurses visit schools to check on the wellbeing of pupils. Responsibilities include detection of poor growth, parasitic infestations and non-accidental injury and promoting vaccination.

Schultze expulsion of the placenta the fetal surface of the placenta appears first at the

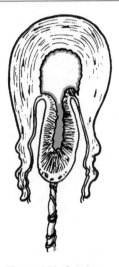

■ **Figure 120** Schultze expulsion of the placenta

vulva during the third stage of labour, as opposed to the maternal surface (*see* Matthew Duncan expulsion and Figure 120).

sciatic nerve a nerve which runs down the back of the leg from the spine.

sciatica severe pain which results from compression of the sciatic nerve. It follows the pathway of a nerve.

scientific method a systematic, ordered way of collecting information in order to formulate theory and predict relationships.

sclerema hardening of the skin and subcutaneous tissue.

sclerema neonatorum subcutaneous hardening of the tissues of the extremities, often due to hypothermia in newborn infants.

scoliosis curving of the spine, also known as lordosis or kyphosis (*see* Figure 121).

screening a test which can be carried out on a large population of apparently healthy people in order to attempt to detect and thus treat diseases early. The test has to be acceptable, reliable (not too many false-positives or false-negatives) and cost-effective. There is a clear distinction between a screening test, which can give an indication of the likelihood of existence of disease, and a diagnostic test, which can positively detect a disease.

Scriver test a biological test used to detect inborn errors of metabolism including phenylketonuria.

scrotum the sac behind the penis in which the testes are located.

scurvy a disease caused by lack of vitamin C in the diet. The person becomes anaemic, develops mouth ulcers, haemorrhages into the mucous membranes and the skin, and has swollen, painful joints.

sebaceous oily.

sebaceous glands small, oil-producing glands near the surface of the skin.

sebum the oily substance produced by the sebaceous glands.

second degree perineal laceration damage to the pelvic floor, including the perineal skin and muscle layers, sustained during the birth of a baby.

second stage of labour the period of labour from the complete dilation of the cervix until the complete birth of the infant. It lasts from several minutes up to 3 hours.

secondary an event which occurs after the main event; not the primary event.

secondary areola development of an extended pigmented area around the areola occurring in pregnancy.

secondary postpartum haemorrhage excessive bleeding

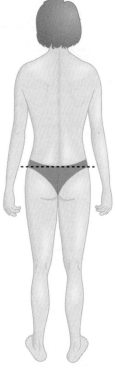
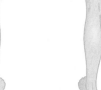

■ **Figure 121** Scoliosis

from the genital tract commencing 24 hours and up to 6 weeks after delivery of the baby, usually due to infection or retained products of conception.

secretion a substance produced by a gland.

secretory phase the second half of the menstrual cycle, after the ovum has been released approximately 14 days before the menses. The corpus luteum increases production of progesterone bringing about glandular

activity in the endometrium and a receptive state for the fertilized ovum (*see* Figure 122).

sedative a drug given to induce deep relaxation and reduce anxiety.

segment a part of the whole. *Upper segment of the uterus* – the body of the uterus responsible for contracting and thickening in labour. *Lower segment of the uterus* – the lower third of the uterus and the cervix, which relaxes and dilates in labour.

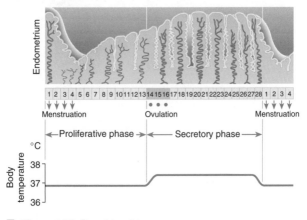

■ Figure 122 Secretory phase

segmentation the process of dividing the whole into parts similar to the whole.

seizure a convulsion or epileptic fit.

self-awareness the development of understanding of one's own beliefs, biases, previous experiences and attitudes and conscious insight into how these can affect one's philosophy and approach to people and practice.

self-concept the image of self, including attitudes that a person holds in their mind.

self-conscious being aware of oneself and one's likely reactions, feelings and desires.

self-esteem the degree of worth one attributes to oneself.

self-governing trust a hospital which has opted out of NHS control and runs its own finances, personnel, etc. It is run by an executive board and a non-executive board but the secretary of state appoints the chairman.

self-help group a collection of lay people with similar interests who meet together to discuss and support one another.

Sellick's manoeuvre the procedure of applying pressure on the cricoid cartilage of the larynx to occlude the oesophagus in order to prevent regurgitation of stomach contents during intubation.

semen the fluid from the prostate gland containing sperm which is ejaculated from the penis during intercourse.

semi- prefix meaning half or partial.

semiconscious a state in which the person is not fully alert or aware of their surroundings.

semipermeable allowing some substances through but not all. The placenta and membranes are semipermeable, allowing some viruses, drugs and alcohol to pass through to the fetus.

semiprone lying on one side with the topmost thigh and arm flexed and forward.

semirecumbent reclining position, half sitting up.

senile vaginitis age-related degeneration of the vagina in which the tissues become less vascular, less elastic and dryer;

may occur post menopausally as the levels of oestrogen secretion fall.

senna (Senokot®) a laxative manufactured from the cassia plant. It can cause abdominal discomfort.

sensation a feeling, impression or awareness of one's physical and emotional state.

sensitive reacting to a stimulus.

sensitization an immunological response occurring after initial exposure of a person to an antigen. The preparation of an organ, e.g. the uterus by bathing it in a hormone such as prostaglandin so that it will respond to another hormone such as oxytocin, triggering contraction and the start of labour.

sensory referring to the senses or sensation.

sensory nerves nerves that detect pressure, pain and temperature and relay this stimulus to the brain for interpretation.

separation anxiety the stress symptoms exhibited by an infant when removed from her or his mother or main carer or when approached by a stranger.

sepsis infection; the presence of harmful organisms where they can cause tissue damage. *Puerperal sepsis* is infection of the genital tract after delivery.

septal defect a congenital abnormality in the wall which divides the left and right sides of the heart, frequently a fistula.

septic the presence of infection.

septic abortion an abortion following which an infection occurs in the uterus, sometimes due to the use of unclean instruments. It can be life-threatening.

septicaemia bacteria in the blood. The person will be very ill, with pyrexia, nausea, vomiting, rigors, headache, joint pains and general malaise.

septum an anatomical structure which divides an organ or tube

in half. The left and right side of the heart are divided by a septum. An unusual uterine anomaly is a septum descending from the fundus which may go through to the vagina or terminate just below the fundus forming a bicornuate uterus.

septuplets seven babies in the uterus or being born at the same time.

sequela (PLURAL sequelae) that which follows or results from something. Referring to a lifelong condition which may follow and be caused by childbirth.

seroconversion the change seen in a series of blood/serology tests, such as antibodies developing in response to a vaccine or infection.

serology the use of antigen/antibody reactions in the laboratory to diagnose infection in blood taken from clients.

serous fluid any fluid resembling serum.

serous membrane a thin but strong sheet of cells which lines cavities. The thoracic and abdominal cavities are lined by two such membranes between which serous fluid is produced, enabling the membranes to move against each other without friction.

serum the yellow sticky fluid left when the cells have been removed from blood.

serum albumin one of the main proteins in the blood which is responsible for its viscosity and maintenance of blood pressure.

serum bilirubin (SBR) the presence in the blood of bilirubin, the product of red cell (erythrocyte) breakdown. Found in the blood of neonates with physiological jaundice. The level is monitored by taking blood from a heel prick and phototherapy is offered if levels are high. High levels can cause staining of the medulla of the brain – kernicterus – and irreversible damage.

sex (gender) species are divided into male and female depending on which gametes they have.

sex chromosome termed the X and Y chromosomes; the genetic component in determining gender.

sex hormones endocrine hormones such as androgens and oestrogens produced by the testes or ovaries that are responsible for influencing development of sexual characteristics.

sex-linked genes refers to the genes which are found only on the sex chromosomes. Some diseases are sex-linked, e.g. haemophilia.

sexism behavioural characteristics of prejudice or discriminatory belief that one gender is superior to another.

sextuplets six babies resulting from one conception.

sexual abuse the forcing upon a person of sexual acts or practices against their will and without their consensual participation.

sexual health freedom from sexually transmitted disease and ability to enjoy sexual expression.

sexual intercourse the physical process during which the erect penis is introduced into the vagina and semen is ejaculated. Sperm in the semen are able to pass through the cervix and swim towards the fallopian tubes in search of an ovum with which to unite.

sexually transmitted disease (STD) diseases such as infection with *Chlamydia trachomatis*, HIV, syphilis and gonorrhoea, which can be passed on during sexual intercourse.

shared care a system whereby the woman receives antenatal care in a collaborative format both from the midwife

(sometimes in her family doctor's surgery) and from a doctor in a hospital or other clinical setting.

sharps used scalpels and needles which are able to cause a laceration or puncture wound and possibly transmit disease to the injured person.

sheath (SYNONYM condom) the rubber tube which is put over the erect penis before penetration during sexual intercourse. It prevents the sperm entering the female body and so avoids conception.

Sheehan's syndrome hypoxia and pituitary necrosis following severe intrapartum conditions such as abruptio placentae or postpartum haemorrhage which can cause shock. Pituitary function is impaired and secondary infertility may ensue.

Shirodkar operation surgical procedure performed at around 16 weeks' gestation where the cervix is deemed 'incompetent'. A purse-string suture is put around the neck of the cervix to keep it closed and in an attempt to prevent abortion (*see* Figure 123).

Shirodkar suture the purse-string suture which is inserted into the cervix during a Shirodkar operation (*see* Figure 123).

shivering involuntary contraction of the tiny muscles under the skin in order to generate heat when cold or in response to fear.

shock a physical state characterized by sudden fall in blood pressure, rapid pulse, abnormal breathing patterns, pallor and loss of full consciousness. Severe shock can be potentially life-threatening.

shoulder dystocia an emergency situation occasionally occurring in the second stage of labour. The head of the baby is born and no further advance

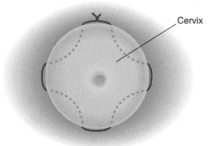

Cervix

■ **Figure 123** Shirodkar suture

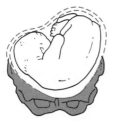

■ **Figure 124** Shoulder presentation

takes place as the shoulders are wedged above the brim of the pelvis.

shoulder presentation the shoulder is presenting over the cervix (*see* Figure 124). This is incompatible with vaginal delivery and labour is obstructed. A caesarean section is usually offered on diagnosis.

show (SYNONYM operculum) the mucoid plug expelled from the cervical canal as the cervix starts to efface and dilate (*see* Figure 125).

shunt the re-routing or bypassing of an organ by an abnormal anatomical opening, e.g. the ductus arteriosus causes blood to bypass the lungs.

SI units (Système International d'Unités; International System of Units) an internationally agreed scale of measurement used in science, industry and pharmaceuticals. It uses metres, kilograms and seconds. (*See* Appendix.)

Siamese twins (SYNONYM conjoined twins) incomplete cleavage of a single fertilized ovum; two babies develop but are anatomically joined at some point.

siblings one, two or more children having the same parents; blood relatives.

sickle cell anaemia a chronic incurable anaemia caused by homozygosity to haemoglobin S. The abnormal haemoglobin makes the erythrocytes very fragile and susceptible to alteration in shape, sometimes triggering a sickle cell crisis.

sickle cell crisis alteration in shape of erythrocytes when the tension (concentration) of oxygen in the cells falls. They are unable to absorb as much oxygen. The loss of discoid shape causes the cells to clump or stick together and so obstruct blood vessels resulting in ischaemia. Severe joint pain,

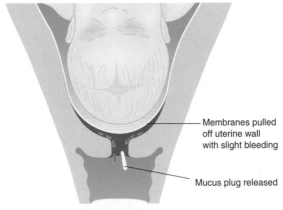

Membranes pulled
off uterine wall
with slight bleeding

Mucus plug released

At start of labour

■ **Figure 125** 'Show'

headaches, dizziness, convulsions, visual disturbances, facial nerve paralysis, breathlessness, cyanosis and shock may result.

sickle cell disease a disease caused by abnormally shaped erythrocytes. Sickle cell crises will occur when the person is stressed. Anaemia is common.

sickle cell trait the Hb S gene has been inherited from one parent. The carrier may have some haemoglobin S but no signs or symptoms of the disease.

side-effect a secondary and undesirable reaction accompanying the desired effect of a drug given with therapeutic intent.

SIDS (sudden infant death syndrome) death of a baby for no apparent reason. Previously called 'cot death'.

sign an indication; something visible, objective.

sigmoid S-shaped region of the large intestine/colon.

significance having an uncertainty of meaning; statistical probability that a given finding may have occurred by chance alone.

Silver–Anderson score a score 0–10 used in preterm infants to measure the degree of respiratory distress they are experiencing. Five aspects are measured: chest retraction on inspiration, intercostal retraction, xiphoid retraction, flaring of the nares and expiratory grunts.

silver nitrate an anti-infective agent historically used in eye drops to prevent gonococcal ophthalmia neonatorum.

Simmonds's disease hypoactivity of the pituitary gland causing all other endocrine glands to be underactive.

Sims's position similar to left lateral but nearer prone.

Sims's speculum a metal instrument used for visualizing the vagina and cervix.

sinciput the brow or the forehead of the fetus; the region found between the coronal suture and orbital ridges.

Singers' test a blood test which indicates whether blood loss is of fetal or maternal origin.

singleton denotes the presence a single fetus in the uterus throughout pregnancy.

skeletal system the combined structure of bones and cartilage providing the protective frame and structure for the body and enabling movement.

Skene's ducts the largest of the urethral glands in the female. They provide lubrication and are equated to the prostate gland in the male.

skull the bony cap over the top of the brain. It comprises three regions: the vault, the face and the base.

small for gestational age (SGA) a fetus that is smaller than expected for its gestation. Detection (by palpation and ultrasound) is important because the fetus is at risk of hypoxia in labour and postnatal problems.

smear a small sample of superficial cells are removed from the cervix to detect hormonal levels and early malignant changes.

smoking in pregnancy toxic substances such as nicotine and carbon dioxide found in cigarettes cause vasoconstriction and reduce the oxygen-carrying capacity of the blood. The fetus receives a reduced supply of nutrients and oxygen which can cause growth retardation.

social class a system used to divide people into categories based on socioeconomic means. The point on which a person is located on the continuum is indicated by occupation. The five demarcations are: professional (I), intermediate (II), skilled (III), semi-skilled (IV) and unskilled (V).

social fund the money set aside by the government to support women and children with no financial resources other than benefits, family credit and income support.

social network a grouping of people with common interests who willingly interact together with mutual benefits.

social services department the government department which is concerned with the welfare of the low income families and those with special needs, disabilities and long-term diseases.

social worker a person trained to assess social need and direct people to appropriate resources. There is a responsibility towards vulnerable members of society, children, the elderly and the homeless.

socioeconomic status the position of an individual on a scale determined by wealth, health and education.

sociology the study of society and how it functions.

sonogram the image obtained by ultrasound scan.

sonography ultrasonography.

souffle a soft blowing sound heard over the abdomen in pregnancy. A *uterine souffle* is the pulsating sound of the uterine arteries.

soya milk a substitute food made from soya beans for babies who cannot tolerate cows' or breast milk.

Spalding's sign the overlapping of the bones of the cranium seen on X-ray examination after fetal death.

spasm an involuntary and uncontrollable movement in a muscle. It is not under the control of the brain.

spastic refers to limb movements which are not under the control of the will/brain. Usually due to cerebral palsy.

special care baby unit (SCBU) a department set up

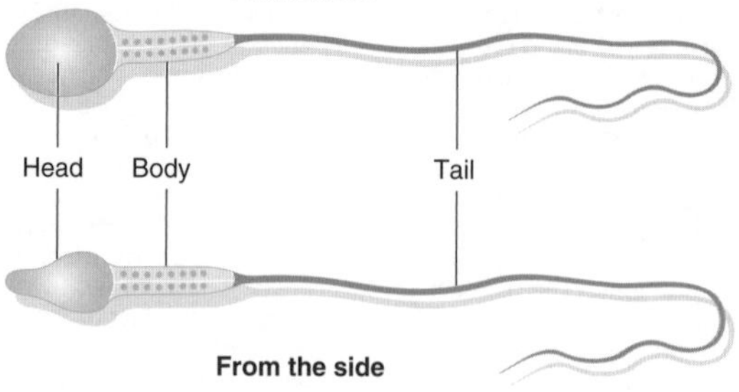

From above

Head   Body   Tail

From the side

■ **Figure 126** Spermatozoa

with equipment and staff to care for the particular needs of babies born preterm or otherwise in poor health. They usually have an intensive care unit attached which specializes in babies needing ventilation.

specific gravity refers to the weight of a fluid compared to water using the same volume. The specific gravity of water is 1000 while urine may be 1010 or more depending on its concentration.

specimen a small sample of the whole; tests can be performed on samples to diagnose the well-being of the whole.

speculum an instrument used to inspect a cavity not usually visible, e.g. the cervix can be seen by inserting a speculum in the vagina.

Spencer Wells artery forceps a type of artery forceps used in surgical procedures.

spermatic referring to sperm.

spermatic cord comprises arteries, nerves and the tube along which sperm pass from the testes to reach the penis.

spermatozoa mature reproductive cells. They are 1/500 inch long, have a head with a nucleus, a neck and a tail for propulsion (*see* Figure 126).

spermicide a cream or gel which is destructive to sperm.

sphincter a strong, round band of muscle fibres which closes or opens a tube or cavity, e.g. the *pyloric sphincter*, the *cardiac sphincter* in the stomach, or the *anal sphincter* which closes the rectum.

sphingomyelin a complex molecule of fat and protein found in the amniotic fluid and measured as a comparative ratio to lecithin to assess fetal lung maturity.

sphygmomanometer an instrument used to measure blood pressure.

spina bifida congenital abnormality of the central nervous system. The bony cavity around the spinal cord is not completely closed and so the meninges herniate through. In severe cases the spinal cord is partially exposed (*see* Figure 127).

spinal refers to the spine.

spinal anaesthetic (SYNONYM spinal block) the dura around the spinal cord is pierced and local anaesthetic is introduced into the cerebrospinal fluid. The sensory nerves are blocked for a short period of time.

spinal headache a severe headache following an epidural

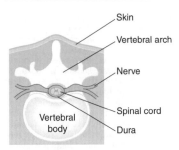
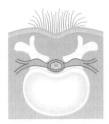

Normal

Oculta spina bifida

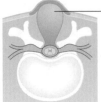

Cerebrospinal fluid

Cerebrospinal fluid and nerve cells

Meningocele

Meningomyolocele

■ **Figure 127** Spina bifida

anaesthetic, lumbar puncture or spinal block caused by the escape of cerebrospinal fluid during the procedure. The headache and accompanying visual disturbances may last several days.

spine the bones of the back that make up the vertebrae and enclose the spinal cord.

spinous process small projections of bony tissue found mainly on the spinal column.

spirochaete a group of microorganisms which appear spiral under a microscope; they cause syphilis.

splint a solid board used to hold the joints either side of a fracture in place or to immobilize an arm if there is an intravenous infusion in place.

spontaneous resulting from natural impulses; happening without intervention.

spontaneous abortion the natural loss of a pregnancy before it is viable.

spontaneous labour the birthing process from the beginning to the end without recourse to mechanical or pharmacological help.

spontaneous vaginal delivery (SVD) delivery of a baby through the vagina without recourse to forceps or ventouse.

spurious labour a false labour.

squamous epithelium the thin fish-like scaley appearance of the cells lining the mouth and vagina.

squatting a position adopted for birth in which the woman crouches close to the ground (*see* Figure 128). A variation of this is the supported squat in which the woman stands with her hips and knees completely flexed supporting herself on her arms or being supported by another. The dimensions of the pelvic outlet are enlarged.

standard a measure which forms the basis of other similar phenomena, values, substances or against which they can be compared or judged. A standard is a predetermined criterion or description of care, used to provide guidance, and can be a measure by which high quality care and professional performance are assessed.

standard deviation a mathematical statement used to describe the dispersion of a set of values or scores from the mean value or score. Each value is subtracted from the mean, squared and the squares are summed. The square root or the summed squares give a mathematically standardized value so that deviations in the sample can be compared.

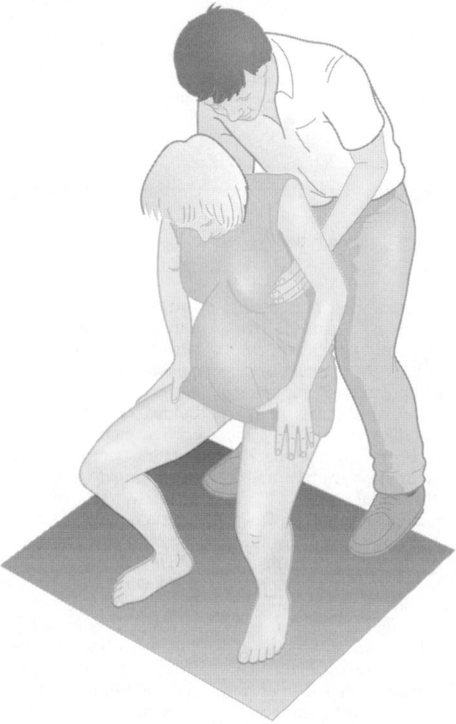

■ **Figure 128** Squatting

standard of care written statement explaining what a person can expect from the professionals around them and by which the professional's performance can be measured.

staphylococci (SINGULAR staphylococcus) a group of pus-forming bacteria which look like a bunch of grapes under a microscope; they can cause puerperal sepsis, urinary tract infections, skin infections and sore throats.

staples small U-shaped pieces of wire used to hold the edges of a skin wound together after surgery and until healing has occurred.

startle reflex (SYNONYM Moro reflex) an involuntary spasmodic movement of the limbs of the infant in response to a sudden stimulus. Used to assess neonates. The head is allowed to drop back; the arms will swing out and return to their mid-line flexed position in a series of jerks. Disturbance in the pattern may indicate neurological damage.

stasis loss of peristaltic movement. *Intestinal stasis* causes constipation and after surgery paralytic ileus (in which the gut is temporarily paralysed).

stat. (LATIN, *statim*) abbreviation used in prescribing medicines meaning given at once, immediately.

State Certified Midwife (SCM) a person who has been trained and deemed competent by the state/government to practise the skills expected of a midwife. Now called a Registered Midwife (RM).

station refers to the position of the fetal head in relation to the ischial spine (*see* Figure 129). It can be assessed on vaginal examination.

statistical significance the interpretation of data suggesting that results arose from a known factor and not simply by chance.

statistics figures and numbers which lead to the postulation of facts and theories.

status epilepticus a rapid succession of epileptic fits with no time for recovery between.

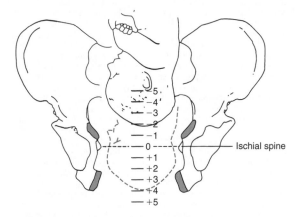

■ **Figure 129** Stations of the fetal head

statutory referring to legislation by parliament.

statutory bodies the organizations set up by parliament in the Nurses, Midwives and Health Visitors Act 1979 to oversee the conduct, practice, training, regulation, register and disciplining of midwives, nurses and health visitors.

statutory maternity pay (SMP) the amount of money paid to a woman during the time she is not at work due to pregnancy or childbirth.

statutory sick pay (SSP) money paid to women on lower incomes who are unable to work due to sickness for more than 4 days before the 28th week of pregnancy.

Stein–Leventhal syndrome a group of symptoms including amenorrhoea, oligomenorrhoea, hirsutism, infertility, polycystic ovaries and high levels of testosterone.

stem cells master cells which develop a few days after fertilization of the ovum. They contain enzymes which enable rapid cell replication and have the capacity to develop into many different specialized tissue cells, e.g. blood, skin, muscle, nerves, etc.

stenosis narrowing, contraction, usually of a muscle. *Pyloric stenosis* is when the sphincter muscle which closes the lower part of the stomach hardens and food cannot pass through. This may be congenital. Surgical correction will be offered.

stereotype a particular view, belief or assumption attributed to a person or group of people based on external characteristics.

sterile 1. unable to conceive children. 2. without the presence of micro-organisms or spores.

sterilization 1. the process by which an object becomes totally free from microbes. 2. surgical procedure to ligate the fallopian tubes or the vas deferens (vasectomy) so that fertilization cannot occur.

sternum bone at the centre front of the ribs, the breast bone.

steroids a group of different hormones with the same basic chemical structure produced mainly by the adrenal cortex and the gonads. Artificially administered, they are used to reduce inflammation not caused by infection.

stethoscope an instrument with ear pieces and tubule for amplification used to auscultate the heart and other sounds within the body. A fetal stethoscope is a trumpet-shaped instrument which when placed over the maternal abdomen will detect the sound of the fetal heart.

stillbirth (SB) a baby born after 24 weeks' gestation which after complete expulsion from its mother has shown no sign of life.

stillbirth certificate a certificate issued by the midwife or doctor present at the birth of a stillborn baby and after examination of the baby. The certificate is given to the parents to enable registration of the birth and obtaining a burial certificate. This statutory duty is usually performed by a doctor but a midwife can and will do it in the absence of a doctor.

stimulate to bring about action. The midwife may stimulate a newborn infant to breathe for the first time.

stimulus anything which causes a person or an organ to respond or become more active than previously; may refer to some drugs.

stomach the sac-like structure at the end of the oesophagus just below the diaphragm into which food passes after being swallowed and in which further digestion occurs.

stool discharge from the rectum.

strabismus a squint, a congenital abnormality of the eyes. One eye appears to look one way while the other eye looks elsewhere.

straight sinus a blood vessel found at the junction of the falx cerebri and the tentorium cerebelli within the skull (*see* Figure 130). In conditions associated with abnormal moulding of the fetal skull it may rupture causing internal haemorrhage and resultant morbidity or mortality.

strawberry mark a congenital mark usually red and caused by a cluster of capillaries near the surface of the skin. It usually fades.

streptococcus (PLURAL streptococci) small, round-shaped bacteria common in the environment and harboured in the throat and nose. Some strains like beta-haemolytic streptococci can cause scarlet fever, tonsillitis and severe puerperal sepsis.

stress tension of the body or mind. If the tension is excessive or prolonged physical or mental dysfunction will occur.

stress test stimulation of the uterus with a small amount of intravenous oxytocin until contractions have been achieved. The baby is monitored for response to the contractions as an indicator of its well-being and predictive ability to withstand labour.

striae gravidarum ('stretch marks') marks over the abdomen, breasts and thighs which can develop during pregnancy as the collagen fibres in the skin tear. They are red at first and fade to silver.

strip membranes vaginal examination whereby a finger is inserted through the cervical os and the amnion and chorion are separated from the lower segment of the uterus. This may stimulate the release of oxytocin and prostaglandins and initiate the start of labour.

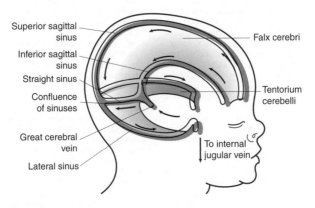

■ **Figure 130** Straight sinus

sub- prefix meaning beneath, under or below.

subarachnoid below the arachnoid mater (membrane), one of the meninges lining the brain and spinal cord.

subarachnoid space not a real space but the area between the arachnoid and the pia mater in which the cerebrospinal fluid circulates.

subarachnoid haemorrhage bleeding into the subarachnoid space.

subclavian beneath the clavicle.

subclavian artery main artery which supplies blood to the arm.

subcutaneous under the skin, into the tissue below the skin.

subcutaneous adipose tissue the fat deposits under the skin.

subcuticular suture a method of bringing together two surfaces by placing a continuous suture beneath the skin along the whole length of the wound. It cannot be seen on the surface and may be more comfortable for the woman than intermittent sutures.

subdural under the dura mater (the membrane surrounding the brain and spinal cord).

subdural haemorrhage bleeding under the dura mater; also called intracranial haemorrhage. Usually results from a traumatic instrumental delivery.

subfertility failure to conceive after unprotected sexual intercourse for more than 1 year (some authorities state 6 months).

subinvolution delay in return of the uterus to its non-pregnant size. This may be due to retained products, infection or caesarean section.

subjective information or experiences as perceived by one person.

sublingual refers to the area under the tongue. A drug can be placed under the tongue where it dissolves and is absorbed by the mucous membranes.

subluxation partial dislocation of a joint or occasionally a ligament.

submucous under the mucous membrane.

subnormal less than that expected of the majority of the population.

suboccipitobregmatic a measurement of the fetal head taken from just above the neck posteriorly to the bregma or anterior fontanelle. It is the smallest diameter and presents when the head is well flexed (*see* Figure 131).

subtotal hysterectomy removal of the body of the uterus, but the cervix and ovaries remain.

succenturiate additional, accessory.

succenturiate placenta placenta containing an extra lobe which is not part of the main organ but is supplied with blood from vessels running through the membranes. The lobe can become detached from the main placenta during the third stage of labour and may possibly remain in the uterus contributing to infection or potentially causing haemorrhage.

suck to draw into the mouth by creating a vacuum and negative pressure with the lips and tongue.

sucking blister formation of a small callous pad on the upper or lower lip of a baby which develops after sucking. It may resemble a blister.

sucking reflex the inborn ability of the newborn to suck in response to stimulation.

suckling a child not yet weaned.

sudden infant death syndrome (SIDS) death of a healthy infant for no apparent cause. Most common between

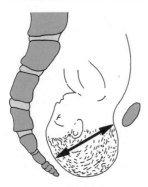

Suboccipitobregmatic 9.5 cm
vertex presentation

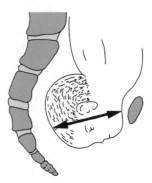

Submentobregmatic 9.5 cm
face presentation

■ **Figure 131** Suboccipitobregmatic

the age of 3 weeks and 6 months and occurring mainly at night, so-called 'cot death'.

sulcus a groove, fold or furrow as between cotyledons of the placenta.

sulphonamides a group of chemicals with a sulphur base used to treat infections especially streptococci, gonococci and *E. coli.*

super-, supra- prefixes meaning over, above or on top of.

superfecundation extra abundant fertility; the fertilization of two ova within the same ovulatory cycle by sperm ejaculated at different times, not necessarily from the same male. The twins will be genetically different.

superfetation fertilization of an ova during a pregnancy. Extremely rare.

superior higher than, above.

superior longitudinal sinus the blood vessel which lies just under the skull bones in the mid-line and passes from front to back.

superior sagittal sinus one of six veins which drain blood

from inside the skull into the jugular vein.

superior vena cava the major blood vessel which takes blood from the upper regions of the body back to the heart.

supervisor of midwives a midwife who has practised for more than 3 years and is appointed by the local supervising authority (LSA) according to rule 44 of the Nurses, Midwives and Health Visitors Rules Approval Order 1986, to be a professional support to all midwives working in her area irrespective of their employer. She will guide, counsel, advise, suggest further development, receive 'Notifications of Intention to Practise', forward them to the LSA, monitor standards of practice, supply orders for drugs, witness destruction of controlled drugs, monitor and store written records, investigate allegations of malpractice and notify the LSA of midwives likely to be a source of infection.

supination of the hand abnormality of the hand in which

it turns upwards. Usually congenital.

supine lying flat on the back.

supine hypotensive syndrome a fall in the blood pressure which occurs when the pregnant woman lies on her back and she experiences a feeling of dizziness on rising. It is due to the gravid uterus compressing the vena cava and reducing venous return to the heart while the woman is supine.

supplement adding to, giving more than is normally available.

supplementary feed additional feed given after a breastfeed; also called a complementary feed.

support groups organizations whose members have common objectives or needs and that are willing to give assistance and encouragement to each other.

suppository medicine formed into a suitable shape which is inserted into the rectum where the drug is absorbed by the mucosa.

suppression to keep down against instinct, impulse or desire.

suppression of lactation prevention of milk secretion by natural methods such as binding or by drugs.

suppuration pus or discharge formation.

suprapubic the region above the pubis bones, found at the front of the abdomen.

suprapubic catheter a urinary catheter inserted through the skin just above the pubic bone following trauma or surgery to the pelvic floor.

surfactant a lipoprotein found in the lungs which keeps the alveoli inflated and reduces surface tension of the pulmonary fluids. It allows exchange of gases in the alveoli and aids the elasticity of pulmonary tissue. Preterm babies lack enough surfactant, making respiration laborious and potentially leading to the development of respiratory distress syndrome.

surgery the branch of medicine which attempts to treat conditions or improve function by means of cutting or operative procedures.

surrogate a person who fulfils the role of another.

surrogate mother a woman who conceives by natural or artificial means with the express intent of giving the child to another woman who is otherwise unable to have babies of her own.

survey a means of discovering information about the population by asking participants to complete a questionnaire or by observing their behaviour.

suture 1. a stitch used to close a wound. 2. membranous lines of indentation found on the fetal skull between two bones where calcification has not yet occurred. They allow moulding to occur in labour and close shortly after birth.

swaddling a method of wrapping a newborn baby that is thought to be comfortable and maintain warmth.

sweat test a method of diagnosing cystic fibrosis early in life. An area of skin is covered and sweating is induced. The sweat is collected and the salt levels analysed. Levels are raised three to six times above the normal in cystic fibrosis.

swimming reflex the innate ability of the infant to temporarily suspend respiration and make swimming movements when placed under water.

sympathetic showing a shared emotional understanding of another's problems and feelings.

sympathetic nervous system that part of the nervous system which prepares the body for 'fight or flight' by increasing the pulse, metabolic rate and blood pressure, dilating the pupils and slowing intestinal peristalsis.

symphysiotomy the cutting of the symphysis pubis to increase the pelvic diameters so that a large baby can pass through the pelvis (*see* Figure 132). It is not performed in the UK.

symphysis that part of the pelvic girdle made of strong cartilaginous tissue which lies between the pubic bones. It softens in pregnancy and increases the pelvic diameters.

symphysis pubis dysfunction (SPD) excessive softening of the cartilage with softening of the pubic bones and destabilization of the joint. Postnatal recovery is slow and not assured.

symptom evidence of a condition or disease presented by the client.

sympus malformation of the feet in which extremities are fused or rotated.

syn-, sym- prefix meaning together.

synclitism when the fetal head enters the pelvis straight, with both parietal bones level with the brim.

syncope loss of consciousness or fainting sometimes due to anaemia.

syncytiotrophoblast the multinucleated protoplasmic substance that surrounds the trophoblast.

syndactyly having webbing or skin layers between the fingers or toes.

syndrome a group of signs and symptoms which occur together in more than one individual and are distinctive to a particular disease.

synopsis a summary or a brief review, a précis.

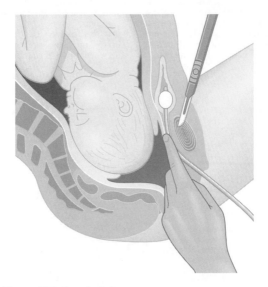

■ **Figure 132** Symphysiotomy

synthesis 1. the binding together of substances not usually found together to form a compound. 2. the linking of previously analysed ideas or concepts to create new ideas, concepts or theories.

synthetic made artificially; not natural.

Syntocinon® (oxytocin) a synthesized drug which causes rhythmic contractions of the uterus. It may be given as a bolus in the third stage of labour to hasten the process or administered as a dilute infusion in the first and second stage of labour and titrated such that contractions occur every 3 minutes.

Syntometrine® a mixture of two drugs, 0.5 mg ergometrine and 5 units of oxytocin (in 1 ml). It is given to women who prefer to have a medically-managed third stage rather than a natural, physiological third stage. In this case it may be given with the birth of the shoulders or after the complete birth of the baby; the latter prevents the possibility of injuring an undiagnosed second twin. It

may also be given to treat post-partum haemorrhage.

syphilis an infectious venereal disease caused by the organism *Treponema pallidum*. It may cross the placental barrier in pregnancy and can cause abortion, stillbirth or congenital syphilis. All pregnant women are offered screening at booking. The infection is effectively treated with penicillin.

Système International d'Unités (International System of Units; SI units) an internationally agreed scale of measurement used in science, industry and pharmaceuticals. It uses metres, kilograms and seconds. (*See* Appendix.)

systemic referring to the whole of the body.

systole the contraction of the heart.

systolic relating to cardiac systole.

systolic murmur abnormal sound heard when the heart contracts.

systolic pressure the pressure exerted on the walls of the arteries when the heart contracts.

Tt

T cell a special lymphocyte made in the bone marrow which matures in the thymus gland and is responsible for immunity and delayed hypersensitivity. The helper cell is a type of T cell responsible for formation of antibodies by B cells.

T-4 cell helper cells secrete interleukin-2 and stimulate production of natural killer cells, gamma interferon, and the suppressor T-8 cells. Human immunodeficiency virus can attack T-4 cells resulting in the body's defences being severely damaged and enabling opportunistic infections to flourish.

TAB a vaccine offering partial protection against typhoid and paratyphoid (A and B) fever.

tablet medicine prepared as a small solid pellet or disc which is usually taken orally and absorbed through the intestinal tract.

tabula rasa describes the mind of a child at birth as blank, clean or empty.

tachycardia fast heart rate.

tachypnoea fast respiratory rate.

tactile relating to touch, feeling a person or object with hands.

tail of Spence the upper outer segment of breast tissue found in the axilla.

talipes (club foot) the foot is bent inwards at birth (*see* Figure 133). It may be caused by the position adopted in the uterus or be due to bone deformity.

talipomanus club hand.

talus the ankle bone.

tampon a wad of cotton wool or cloth with a thread or tape

Talipes equinovarus

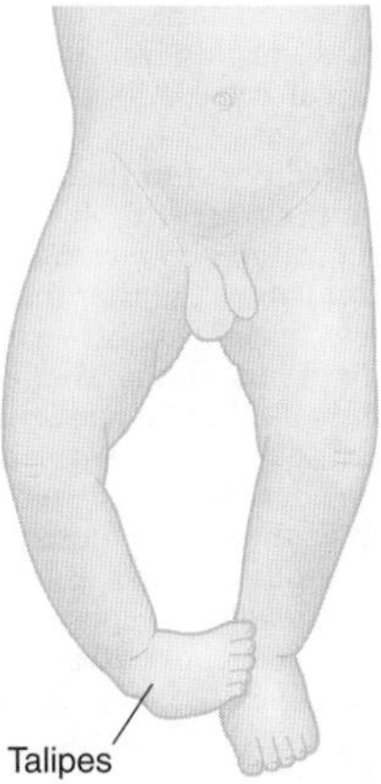

■ **Figure 133** Talipes (club foot)

attachment; inserted into the vagina to absorb menstrual discharge.

tantrum a sudden display of anger usually caused by frustration; common in children aged about 2 years.

tarsus the seven bones of the ankle which allow the foot to rotate in all directions.

taurine a substance present in bile, it combines with cholic acid to make bile salts and enables conjugation of bilirubin.

Taussig–Bing syndrome an abnormal development of the heart in which there is transposition of the main vessels, accompanied by ventricular septal defect and ventricular hypertrophy.

Tay–Sachs disease an inherited neurodegenerative disorder of lipid metabolism caused by a deficiency of the enzyme hexosaminidase A. It is found among Ashkenazi Jews and can be detected antenatally by a maternal blood test. It causes progressive mental and physical retardation and early death.

TBA (traditional birth attendant) definition applied by health organizations to a woman who accompanies another and provides psychological support throughout labour. The term is mainly used in underdeveloped countries. These women are often described as midwives within their own community and by other midwives who feel that midwifery expertise does not have to come from an institutionally-based and nationally-recognized programme to be valid.

t.d.s. (LATIN, *ter die sumendus*) instruction to give the prescribed medicine three times a day.

tea tree oil an aromatic essential oil thought to have antibacterial, antifungal, antimicrobial and antiviral properties.

team midwifery a small group of midwives offer total care to a designated group of pregnant women throughout their entire childbearing experience.

teething the eruption of teeth from the gums.

telangiectatic naevus a flat pink/purple area seen on the skin of the neonate where capillary dilation has occurred. Usually found on the back of the neck or head, eyelids, nose or upper lip.

telemeter the recording and transmission of information by radio waves to a distal base station. The fetal heart can be monitored using this technology.

telemetry the recording of fetal heart rate and contractions by remote control.

temperament a personality type – happy, free and easy, melancholy, etc.; may indicate how a woman will cope with pain in labour and adapt to motherhood.

temperature the amount of heat in the body. Normal temperature is between 36 and 37°C. Babies' temperatures can vary from 35.5°C to 37.5°C, the wide variation being due to an immature physiological mechanism.

temporal refers to the side part of the skull.

temporal bones the bones situated above the ear.

tenacious maintaining a firm hold, sticky, e.g. secretions such as mucus from the vagina.

tendon strong connective tissue which links a bone to a muscle.

TENS (transcutaneous electrical nerve stimulation) a method of pain relief used in labour. It is of uncertain physiology but may work by triggering release of natural endorphins and enkephalins or by blocking (gate control theory) transmission of pain stimulus to the brain.

tension two forces exerting pressure in opposite directions.

tentorium cerebelli the fold of dura mater which extends horizontally inside the skull and separates the cerebral hemispheres from the cerebellum.

tepid slightly warm, up to 32°C.

ter in die (t.i.d.) used of medicine, meaning administer three times a day.

teras a malformed fetus or infant.

teratogen an agent that will cause fetal abnormalities if ingested or inhaled.

teratoma a congenital growth containing hair, nail or bone in an abnormal site.

term the natural end of pregnancy. Sometimes defined as 280 days or 40 weeks after the first day of the last normal menstrual period, or a period between 37 completed weeks and 42 completed weeks after the first day of the last normal menstrual period.

term infant a neonate born after 37 completed weeks' but before 43 weeks' gestation.

termination of pregnancy (TOP) removal from the uterus of the products of conception surgically and under general anaesthetic before the 12th week of pregnancy or by induction in later pregnancy.

tertiary third stage, as in tertiary syphilis.

test procedure done to confirm or eliminate suggestion of possible disease. A *pregnancy test* is a laboratory procedure done to determine the presence of a pregnancy. *Glucose tolerance test* is a series of examinations of the blood after the person has been given a measured quantity of glucose orally (used to detect diabetes).

test tube baby a term used to describe an infant conceived by introduction of an ovum and sperm in a laboratory and later implanted into the mother's uterus (IVF).

testes (SINGULAR testis; SYNONYM testicles) two glands located in the scrotum which produce spermatozoa and testosterone (*see* Figure 134).

testicles *see* testes.

testicular relating to the testes.

testosterone male sex hormone responsible for male body characteristics and sex drive.

tetanic related to tetanus, the painful tonic muscular spasm.

tetanus a disease caused by an anaerobic organism, *Clostridium tetani*, found naturally in soil. The organism causes spasm of muscles including those involved in respiration.

tetanus toxoid a preparation of detoxified tetanus toxin which will produce an immune response to *Clostridium tetani*.

tetracycline a broad spectrum antibiotic contraindicated in pregnancy. It causes discoloration of the child's teeth and early degeneration of the first teeth.

tetradactyly congenital presence of four digits on hands or feet.

tetralogy collection of four things, as in *Fallot's tetralogy* – four congenital abnormalities affecting the heart: pulmonary stenosis, ventricular septal defect, dextroposition of the aorta and right ventricular hypertrophy.

tetraplegia paralysis of all four limbs.

thalassaemia a haemoglobinopathy found in people of Mediterranean origin; the erythrocytes are abnormally small, pale and fragile. *Thalassaemia major*, the homozygous form, may present with severe haemolytic anaemia in childhood. *Thalassaemia minor* is the heterozygous form of the condition in which there is no clinical evidence of abnormality.

thalidomide a sedative and hypnotic drug formerly given to treat morning sickness but which caused severe limb abnormalities.

theca a capsule or enveloping sheath in which another structure is encased or protected.

theory an idea or a collection of arguable propositions used to explain an occurrence, situation or circumstance.

therapeutic relating to therapy, beneficial treatment.

therapeutic abortion termination of a pregnancy deemed necessary to preserve the health of the mother.

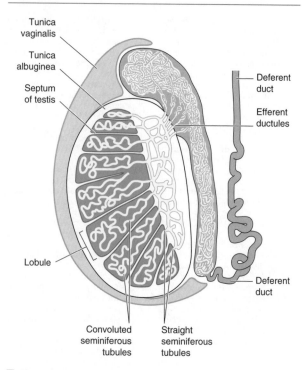

Tunica vaginalis

Tunica albuginea

Septum of testis

Deferent duct

Efferent ductules

Lobule

Deferent duct

Convoluted seminiferous tubules

Straight seminiferous tubules

■ **Figure 134** Testicles

therapy treatment.

thermal refers to the production and maintenance of heat.

thermometer a small glass tube having a hollow vacuumed centre with a small amount of mercury which expands and rises according to the body temperature.

thermoneutral environment conditions designed so that the body temperature can be maintained with the least consumption of oxygen and energy.

thiamine vitamin B₁, part of the vitamin B complex required for neurological and cardiac functioning.

third degree perineal laceration perineal trauma involving skin, muscle and the anal sphincter (*see* Figure 135).

third stage of labour the stage of labour following complete expulsion of the fetus until the placenta and membranes have been delivered and haemorrhage controlled. Physiologically it can take 20–60 minutes, sometimes longer.

thoracic referring to the thorax or chest cavity.

thorax the chest – that part of the body containing the lungs, heart, oesophagus, and bronchi and enclosed by the diaphragm,

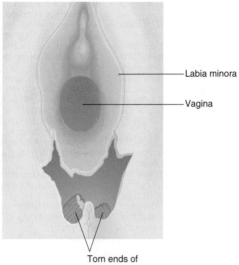

Labia minora

Vagina

Torn ends of
anal sphincter

■ **Figure 135** Third degree perineal laceration (third degree tear)

vertebral column, ribs and sternum.

threatened abortion bleeding in early pregnancy without dilation of the cervix. The bleeding may stop and the pregnancy continue or the cervix may start to dilate making it an inevitable abortion.

threshold the level that must be reached before a certain reaction occurs.

thrill a tremor or vibration transmitted in fluid, felt by tapping the abdomen if polyhydramnios is present.

thrombectomy the surgical removal of a clot of blood from a vessel.

thrombin an enzyme liberated from shed blood that induces clotting by converting the plasma protein fibrinogen into fibrin which forms a clot.

thrombocyte a blood platelet.

thrombocythaemia an abnormally large number of platelets in the blood.

thrombocytopenia an abnormally low number of platelets in the blood, occasionally seen in neonates.

thromboembolism part of a blood clot which has broken off and is circulating in the blood. When it reaches small vessels it can cause a blockage.

thrombophlebitis inflammation of a vein with the formation of a clot; can occur in pregnancy as a result of weight of the uterus on the vessels and sluggish venous return.

thromboplastin the substance liberated from damaged tissues which stimulates clot formation by acting on prothrombin.

thrombosis the formation of a thrombus or clot.

thrombus a clot caused by stasis of blood, usually in a vein.

thrush a fungal infection occurring in the vagina, mouth or sometimes between the toes. It is caused by *Candida albicans*. Neonates may contract it passing through an infected vagina or from the skin of the breast where there is poor hygiene.

thyroid gland found anteriorly at the base of the neck, it straddles the trachea. This endocrine gland secretes thyroxin and tri-iodothyronine which control the metabolic rate. The Guthrie test can detect underactivity of the gland in infants enabling early treatment which prevents cretinism.

t.i.d. (LATIN, *ter in die*) used of medicine, meaning administer three times a day.

tingling prickling or vibrating sensation felt on the skin, usually in the path of a nerve.

tissue a mass of similar cells which act together to perform a specific function.

tissue fluid tiny amounts of fluid around the outside of each cell called extracellular fluid. Too much of this fluid is called oedema. It can occur towards the end of normal pregnancy around the ankles.

titre the amount of a substance administered according to the reaction in the body. Insulin is given in differing amounts according to the changing levels of glucose in the blood. A Syntocinon® infusion is titrated according to the contraction of the uterus, the dose being increased in labour until there are three contractions in 10 minutes or, where necessary, decreased to avoid overstimulation.

toco- a combining form meaning childbirth, derived from the Greek word *tokos* – birth.

tocograph a technique used to record the frequency and amplitude of contractions.

tocolytic a drug used to relax the muscles of the uterus and so stop contractions, e.g. ritodrine hydrochloride (Yutopar®) or salbutamol (Ventolin®).

tocotransducer a piece of electronic equipment used to measure the pressure felt over the abdomen during a uterine contraction.

toddler a child between the age of 1 year and 3 years who is learning to walk and whose maturity and behaviour can be mapped according to a standard pattern.

tolerance the body's ability to respond less aggressively to a substance due to continuous exposure.

tomograph radiological images of soft tissue made at various depths.

tone the amount of tension in a muscle.

tongue tie a congenital abnormality in which there is shortening of the frenulum – the fibrous tissue which anchors the tongue to the base of the mouth.

tonic contractions sustained uterine contractions, lasting longer than a minute thereby reducing placental perfusion to levels which may result in fetal hypoxia.

topical referring to direct application to a mucous membrane or the skin. Topical application comes in the form of a cream, paste, lotion or gel.

top-up additional administration of a substance, intended to elevate a declining level, for instance in epidural anaesthesia. The first 'top-up' injection of analgesic drug through the catheter into the epidural space is done by the anaesthetist. Subsequent top-ups may be administered by a midwife.

TORCH infection a group of infections (including toxoplasmosis, other (syphilis), rubella, cytomegalovirus and herpes) for which the neonate can be screened especially on admission to a special care unit.

torsion twisting; can occur to a tube, e.g. the fallopian tube, a hernia, the testicles, the intestines or a cyst on the end of a stalk.

tort a wrong, breach of contract or act of negligence recognized in and by the law.

tourniquet a tight band of rubber or fabric applied to a limb to arrest haemorrhage or prevent emptying of a vein.

toxaemia toxins or poisons of some description in the blood.

toxic refers to a substance or gas which will cause severe deterioration in health.

toxic shock syndrome an acute bacterial infection caused by *Staphylococcus aureus* and characterized by fever, diarrhoea, erythematous rash and shock. It is thought to be associated with the use of tampons.

toxin a substance which can cause damage to health or congenital abnormalities if exposure should occur during pregnancy.

toxoid a toxin which has been treated with chemicals or heat to render it non-toxic but when introduced to the body can stimulate the production of antibodies.

toxoplasmosis a protozoal infection with influenza-like symptoms. If acquired in early pregnancy the infection can cross the placenta and infect the fetus causing abortion. Acquired in later pregnancy, it can cause multiple abnormalities.

trachea the windpipe, a cartilaginous cylinder which allows air to pass from the larynx to the bronchi.

trachelorraphy an operation to repair a torn cervix.

tracheo-oesophageal fistula a congenital abnormality in which there is a hole enabling communication between the trachea and the oesophagus. Food may pass into the lungs causing choking and air may pass into the stomach.

trait characteristic feature of a disease or personality. A person with *sickle cell trait* has inherited one gene for sickle cell anaemia and can pass it on to his offspring.

traditional birth attendant *see* TBA.

tranquillizer a drug which is used to calm an anxious person.

transcervical ligaments the bands of fibrous tissue which hold the cervix in position and are attached to the lateral walls of the pelvis.

transcutaneous electrical nerve stimulation *see* TENS.

transducer a machine which converts one form of energy into another capable of sending and receiving sound signals. When using ultrasound the transducer transforms electrical energy into vibrations of sound the frequency of which cannot be detected by the ear.

transferrin a serum globulin (protein) that binds and transports iron in the blood.

transfusion introduction of a substance directly into the bloodstream.

transition a state of change; the period towards the end of the first stage of labour and the beginning of the second stage.

translocation the detachment of a part of one chromosome and attachment onto another.

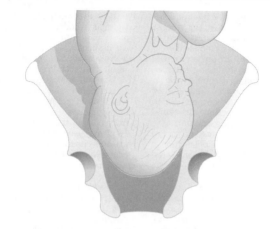

■ **Figure 136** Transverse arrest

transplacental across the placental barrier.

transport movement of material across or into cells.

transposition 1. a congenital abnormality in which one part of the body normally located on the right is found on the left and vice versa. 2. the shifting of genetic material from one chromosome to another. *Transposition of the great vessels* is a congenital heart anomaly in which the pulmonary artery arises from the left ventricle and the aorta from the right ventricle.

transudate fluid with very few particles which squeezes through cells or membranes.

transvaginal through the vagina.

transverse arrest interruption in the passage of the fetal head through the pelvis during labour. Rotation and descent are obstructed, usually by prominent ischial spines (*see* Figure 136).

transverse lie the position of the fetal spine in relation to the mother's spine. The two are at right angles to each other. No presenting part can be identified.

transverse presentation the fetus is lying across the uterus and the inlet of the pelvis.

transverse sinuses a pair of venous sinuses in the tentorium cerebelli under the skull.

trauma 1. sudden injury or damage to the body. 2. an incident which results in physical or emotional injury.

traumatic relating to, caused by trauma.

travail labour or hard work.

Trendelenburg position lying on the back with the body at an angle of 30 degrees and the head at the lowest point.

treponema pallidum the spirochaete which causes syphilis.

trial of labour conducted in circumstances where the fetal head has not engaged in the hope that a vaginal delivery may be possible. Induction of labour may be offered and the woman's progress closely monitored. If progress is not

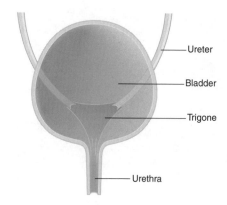

Ureter

Bladder

Trigone

Urethra

■ **Figure 137** Trigone of bladder

maintained a caesarean section will be offered.

trial of scar term used to describe the medical approach to vaginal birth after caesarean, where doubt is thrown on the ability of the scar from the previous caesarean section(s) to withstand labour without dehiscing or rupturing. Separation of scar tissue causes pain and, later, vital signs will deviate from the normal range.

trichomoniasis, trichomonas vaginitis a common vaginal infection caused by a flagellate protozoan. Vaginal discharge may be watery, frothy, yellow/ green.

trigone a triangular area at the base of the bladder between the ureters and the urethral openings (*see* Figure 137). The area is not very elastic. As it lies against the anterior wall of the vagina the trigone may be damaged as the vagina distends in the second stage of labour.

trimester a period of 3 months. In pregnancy there are three trimesters, early, mid and last trimester.

tripartite three partitions or parts of a placenta each joined to the other by the cord.

triple test a maternal blood test performed at approximately 16 weeks' gestation to determine levels of alphafetoprotein, unconjugated oestriol and human chorionic gonadotrophin. These substances are quantified and correlated to the mother's age to calculate her individual risk of the fetus having Down's syndrome.

triple vaccine a combined vaccine against tetanus, diphtheria and pertussis.

triplets three babies in the same pregnancy.

trisomy addition of a single chromosome to another pair, as in *trisomy 18* (Edwards's syndrome), *trisomy 21* (Down's syndrome) and *trisomy 13* (Patau's syndrome).

trocar a sharp, pointed metal instrument fitted inside of a cannula used for puncturing the body.

trochanter one of two bony prominences on the head of the femur bone.

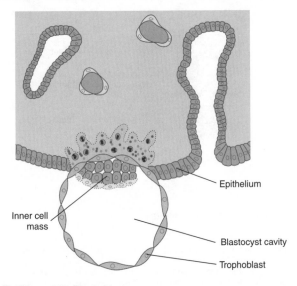

■ **Figure 138** Trophoblast

trophoblast the outer layer of the blastocyst in embryonic life from which the placenta and chorionic membrane develop (*see* Figure 138).

trophoblastic pertaining to the trophoblast, syncytiotrophoblast and cytotrophoblast.

true conjugate refers to the anterior–posterior diameter of the pelvic inlet, taken from the sacral promontory to the centre of the upper surface of the symphysis pubis (*see* Figure 139).

true labour uterine contractions which cause the cervix to dilate – as opposed to contractions which do not result in the birth of a baby.

trust a unit of management within the UK National Health Service, usually a hospital or community area from which GPs can buy services for their clients.

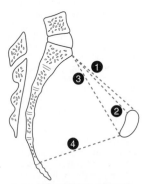

1. Anatomical/'true' conjugate
2. Obstetrical conjugate
3. Internal/diagonal conjugate
4. Obstetrical anterior–posterior of outlet

■ **Figure 139** True conjugate

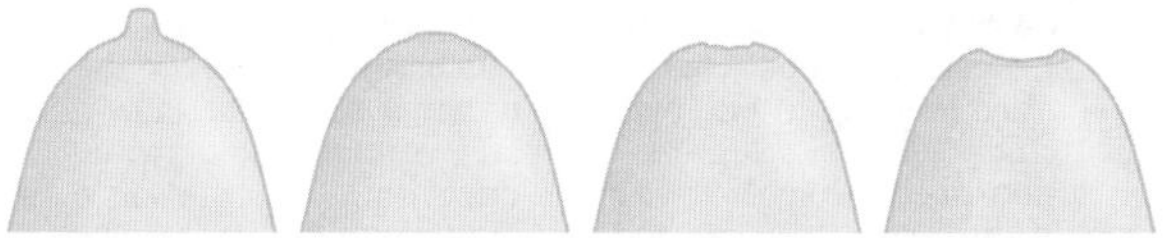

| Normal | Flat | Depressed | Inverted |

■ **Figure 140** Types of nipples

tubal dermoid cyst a tumour containing embryonic tissue growing in an oviduct.

tubal insufflation dilation of the fallopian tubes. Carbon dioxide is pumped into the uterus and expected to pass through the fallopian tubes into the abdominal cavity. On X-ray the gas will be seen under the diaphragm, proving that the fallopian tubes are patent.

tubal ligation surgical tying and cutting of the fallopian tube to prevent any meeting of ova and sperm.

tubal pregnancy development and implantation of the fertilized ovum in the fallopian tube.

tube feeding direct introduction of food into the stomach via the orogastric or nasogastric route.

tuberculosis a notifiable infectious disease transmitted by airborne droplets.

tuberosity the thickened expanded portion of a bone. The *ischial tuberosity* is part of the ischial bone which is thick and upon which the body rests when in the sitting position.

tubo-ovarian abscess a capsule filled with infected material involving the ovary and fallopian tube.

tubo-ovarian cyst a fluid-filled sac involving the ovary and fallopian tube.

tubo-ovarian gestation an ectopic pregnancy which develops between the ovary and the fallopian tube.

tuboplasty surgical repair of the fallopian tube or restructuring

to reverse a tubal ligation and restore fertility.

tubular necrosis death of cells in a tube, e.g. the nephrons, small tubules of the kidney. High blood pressure can cause the epithelial lining of the nephron to be damaged; this may block the nephron or cause release of toxins which will raise the blood pressure.

tubule microscopic tube in the nephron of the kidney.

tunica an enveloping coat of fibrous connective membranes which covers an organ.

tunica albuginea a layer of connective tissue found below the germinal epithelium of the ovary.

tunnel a passage through solid material. The *carpal tunnel* is the passage between wrist bones through which the medial nerve and tendons pass to the hand. *Carpal tunnel syndrome* in pregnancy can occur when oedema causes pressure at this point on the medial nerve. An uncomfortable tingling sensation in the fingers may be felt.

Tuohy needle the blunt needle and cannula used to locate the epidural space around the spine.

Turner's syndrome a congenital abnormality in which there are 45 instead of 46 chromosomes. One of the sex chromosomes is absent so the child will appear female, have a vagina, uterus and fallopian tubes but the ovaries will not function.

twin-to-twin transfusion transfer of blood from one fetus to the other resulting in one twin being polycythaemic, large and well nourished, while the other one is small, hypovolaemic and anaemic. Both babies are at risk of cardiac failure.

twins two babies born from the same pregnancy. They may be identical or non-identical.

types of nipples *normal*: the ducts protrude in the aerola beyond the curve of the breast tissue; *flat*: the ducts are flush with the soft tissue of the breast; *depressed*: the ducts are below the level of the skin of the breast, forming a small saucer shape; *inverted*: the tiny muscles of the erectile tissue are contracted, drawing the ducts down into the soft tissue of the breast. They are likely to be kinked, obstructing the flow of milk (*see* Figure 140).

typhus an acute infectious illness transmitted to humans by rats and lice. Pyrexia, headache, rash and severe malaise will be present. The condition can be fatal.

typing the process of classifying blood tissues and other materials according to the characteristics they share.

Uu

ulcer a lesion on the skin or in the mucous membrane of the mouth or vagina, caused by trauma, infection or pressure on blood vessels. Healing is sometimes slow.

ulna the inner of the long bones in the forearm whose lower process forms the point of the elbow.

ultrasonic sound which cannot be heard with the ear, having in excess of 20 000 cycles per second. A transducer emits short pulses of high frequency sound, these are bounced off structures within the body and the echoes collected and displayed on a cathode ray tube (*see* Figure 141).

ultrasonogram picture of an internal organ produced by ultrasound scanning.

ultrasonography the process of making pictures of the deep structures of the body by measuring and recording the reflection of pulsed or continuous high frequency sound waves.

ultrasound sound waves at a high frequency of over 20 000 kHz. It is used for examining the fetus in utero, for dating, measuring growth, assessing for structural abnormalities and recording the heart rate and reaction to labour. The safety of ultrasound in pregnancy has not been proven and the accuracy of ultrasound in detecting anomalies and dating pregnancy has been questioned.

ultraviolet light rays from the sun with extremely short wavelengths not visible to the human eye. They are grouped by types

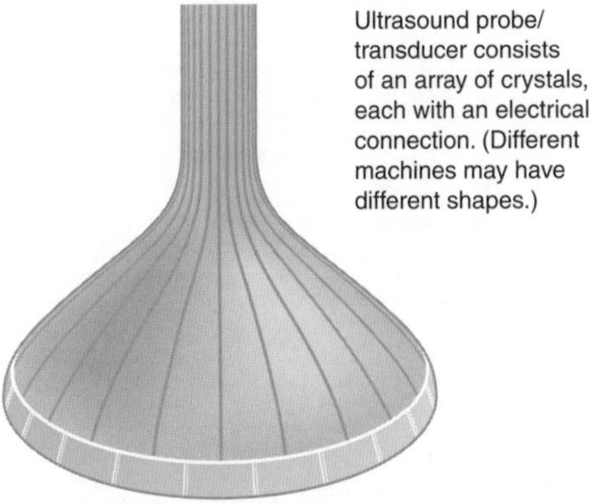

Ultrasound probe/transducer consists of an array of crystals, each with an electrical connection. (Different machines may have different shapes.)

■ **Figure 141** Ultrasound transducer

A, B, C and R according to wavelength and are able to penetrate the skin and cause burns. They are used in phototherapy units for treatment of neonates who are jaundiced. The light helps break down the bilirubin in the skin.

umbilical relating to the umbilicus.

umbilical catheterization the passing of a fine catheter into the vein of the umbilicus and to the liver for purposes of feeding and assessing the condition of a sick neonate.

umbilical cord the cord containing (usually) two arteries and one vein which connects the fetus to the placenta (*see* Figure 142). Anomalies in the number of cord vessels may be indicative of kidney disease.

umbilical cord presentation the membranes are intact but the cord can be felt in front of the fetal head. (*See also* Figure 33.)

umbilical cord prolapse the passage of the cord out of the uterus following rupture of the membranes. It may stay in the vagina or pass beyond the vulva in which case the cold air may cause the vessels to go into spasm stopping blood reaching the fetus. Alternatively the descent of the presenting part may compress the cord. Both situations are obstetric emergencies usually requiring caesarean section. (*See also* Figure 34.)

umbilical hernia protrusion of the small intestines through a weakness in the muscular wall of the abdomen at the umbilicus. The swelling will become smaller as the child grows.

umbilical region area of the abdomen around the umbilicus, middle zone.

umbilical vein one of a pair of vessels through which oxygenated blood passes from the placenta to the fetus.

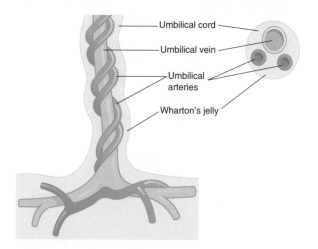

Umbilical cord
Umbilical vein
Umbilical arteries
Wharton's jelly

■ **Figure 142** Umbilical cord

umbilicus the navel – the scar remaining after separation of the umbilical cord.

unconscious totally unaware of surroundings, unresponsive to stimuli.

unengaged head on abdominal examination the fetal head is palpated above the pelvic brim.

uni- prefix meaning one or single.

UNICEF (United Nations International Children's Emergency Fund) a fund set up in 1946 by the United Nations to aid children in devastated areas of the world through provision of food, medical treatment, vaccinations, vitamins and education.

unicellular containing one cell only.

uniform one common distinctive set of clothing worn by all people of the same organization or occupation.

unilateral one side only.

uniovular one ovum (from which identical twins develop).

unisex 1. referring to only one gender. 2. having reproductive organs for one sex only. 3. clothing designed to be worn by both genders.

universal donor a person with blood group O Rh negative who may give blood to any person without risk of a reaction.

universal precautions recommended standard of practice of all clinicians designed to prevent transmission of infectious diseases including HIV and hepatitis. It includes the wearing of protective layers of clothing and cleaning procedures including hand washing.

universal recipient a person with blood group AB Rh positive may receive blood from any person without a reaction.

unstable lie refers to the continuing changing lie of the fetus in utero. It cannot be predicted what the lie will be when labour starts. There is a risk of cord prolapse.

unsupported mother a pregnant woman without a partner to provide psychological or financial support to herself and assist with caring for the child.

upper respiratory tract infection (URTI) includes colds, tonsillitis, pharyngitis, rhinitis and laryngitis.

uraemia the term implies excessive uric acid in the blood. This is a pathophysiological state resulting from renal failure. There is acidosis, disturbance in electrolyte balance, sodium and water retention, oedema and hyperkalaemia.

uranoschisis cleft palate.

uranostaphyloplasty the surgical repair of a cleft palate.

urate salts derived from uric acid, found in blood. They may be deposited in joints and when this is the big toe it is referred to as gout.

urea the excreted product of protein metabolism. It is filtered out of the blood by the kidneys and passed down to the bladder for voiding at a suitable time. Blood urea level is normally 2.5–5.8 mmol/L.

ureter tube which passes from the kidneys to the bladder and carries urine. The effect of high levels of progesterone in pregnancy cause dilation and stasis of urine in the ureters with an increased risk of infection.

ureteric referring to the ureters.

ureteritis inflammation or infection in the ureter.

urethra tube from the bladder to the external orifice through which urine is discharged. It is 20 cm long in the male and 3.5 cm in the female. It can be stretched or bruised during childbirth especially in association with forceps delivery. This can lead to urinary retention and overflow incontinence.

urethral referring to the urethra.

urethral sphincter the voluntary muscle at the neck of the bladder which relaxes during urination.

urethrocele herniation of the wall of the urethra so that it protrudes into the vagina.

urethrocystitis inflammation of the urethra and bladder.

uric referring to urine.

uric acid the product of protein metabolism, found in the blood (0.13–0.42 mmol/L) and urine (less than 1 g/day).

urinalysis physical, biochemical and microscopic examination of the urine to detect abnormalities. During pregnancy urine is examined for glucose to detect intolerance or diabetes, protein to detect pre-eclampsia or infection, ketones to detect dehydration or fat metabolism and blood to detect infection or kidney damage.

urinary related to urine.

urinary frequency the desire to void urine very often.

urinary ileostomy the surgical construction of a passage from the bladder to the ilium, which is then used as a urinary reservoir.

urinary incontinence involuntary passage of urine; the inability to control the bladder sphincter leading to leakage of urine.

urinary retention the state where the bladder cannot be emptied despite the desire to do so. Can occur following forceps delivery, epidural anaesthesia, caesarean section, cases of incarcerated gravid uterus and anterior vaginal wall laceration. The bladder will be palpable abdominally.

urinary tract infection (UTI) bacterial growth in the urinary tract. The presence of pus turns the urine cloudy. Potential complications of UTI include kidney damage and possibly preterm labour.

urination the act of passing urine.

urine the clear, straw-coloured fluid secreted by the kidneys as a result of filtering impurities out of the blood.

urinometer a glass cylinder into which urine is collected and a float deposited, used to measure the specific gravity of the urine.

urobilinogen a colourless compound formed in the intestines after the breakdown of bilirubin and present in urine.

URTI *see* upper respiratory tract infection.

urticaria characteristic reaction in which the skin is raised and itchy.

uterine referring to the uterus.

uterine bruit the sound heard with a stethoscope as blood pulsates through the arteries of the uterus.

uterine prolapse descent of the uterus from its normal location in the vagina due to weakened pelvic floor muscles.

uterine souffle a soft blowing sound heard as the blood passes through the vessels of the placenta.

uterine tetany prolonged uterine contractions.

uteroplacental referring to the junction where the placenta meets the inner lining of the uterus.

uterosacral referring to the uterus and the sacrum.

uterosacral ligament a thick fibrous band connecting the cervix to the sacrum and offering support to the uterus.

uterosalpingography radiological examination of the uterus and fallopian tubes. Radioactive dye is introduced into the uterus and left to track into the fallopian/uterine tube and X-rays are taken to detect defects.

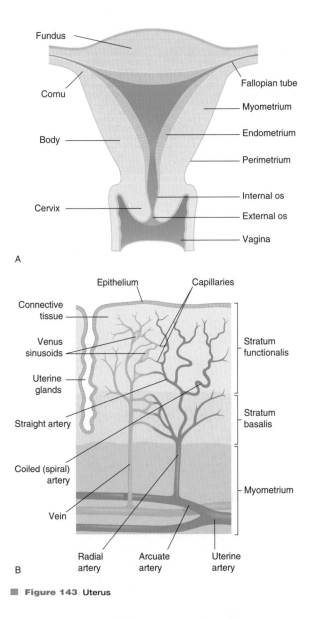

Figure 143 Uterus

uterotomy (SYNONYM hysterotomy) cutting into the uterus.

uterovesical referring to the uterus and the bladder.

uterovesical pouch the fold of peritoneum between the bladder and the uterus.

uterus the womb, the organ which receives and grows the fertilized ovum during development of the fetus and actively participates in its expulsion as part of the birthing process (*see* Figure 143).

uterus bicornis (bicornate uterus) a uterus which divides in two at the upper pole but is fused at the lower pole.

UTI *see* urinary tract infection.

utilitarianism an ethical concept which states that all action should be guided by the desire to bring about the greatest happiness for the greatest number of people.

uvula soft, fleshy pendant hanging from the edge of the soft palate at the back of the mouth.

Vv

vaccinate to inoculate or introduce a vaccine into the body.

vaccination an injection of attenuated (weakened) micro-organisms, bacteria or viruses which may induce immunity or reduce the effects of a disease.

vaccine the suspension of attenuated or killed micro-organisms which is administered during vaccination.

vacuum aspiration 1. withdrawal of substances using negative pressure. 2. termination of an early pregnancy by sucking it out of the uterus through the cervix.

vacuum extraction the delivery of a term baby by applying a suction cap to its scalp. A vacuum is created and traction applied as the mother pushes. This aids her efforts to deliver the baby without recourse to application of forceps.

vagal referring to the vagus nerve.

vagina hollow tube 10 cm long extending from the vulva to the cervix. The lining of squamous epithelium is in folds or rugae which will stretch easily.

vaginal referring to the vagina.

vaginal atrophy postmenopausal condition occurring where oestrogen levels are lowered.

vaginal bleeding may be from a local ulceration of the vagina or from the uterus in pregnancy which is called an antepartum haemorrhage (APH) or threatened abortion, depending on gestation.

vaginal cyst abnormal closed sac or pouch, filled with fluid or connective tissue.

vaginal delivery birth of a fetus through the vagina.

vaginal discharge an emission or secretion that may be clear or pearly-white, containing endocervical cells. If offensive or green it can indicate infection.

vaginal examination (VE) examination per vaginum. The index and middle fingers are passed through the vagina to assess the dilation, thickness and consistency of the cervix, the state of the membranes, the presentation, position and station of the presenting part of the fetus.

vaginal fornix a recess in the upper part of the vaginal canal caused by protrusion of the cervix. Prostin® pessaries are inserted into the posterior fornix.

vaginal hysterectomy removal of the uterus through an incision in the vagina.

vaginal jelly common term applied to a contraceptive product containing a spermicide. Used in conjunction with a contraceptive diaphragm or cervical cap to occlude the cervix and prevent pregnancy occurring.

vaginal lubricant an ointment or cream used to reduce friction in the vagina during intercourse or vaginal examination.

vaginal septum a fold of tissue dividing the length of the vagina (*see* Figure 144). A congenital abnormality caused by incomplete development of the genitalia in embryonic life.

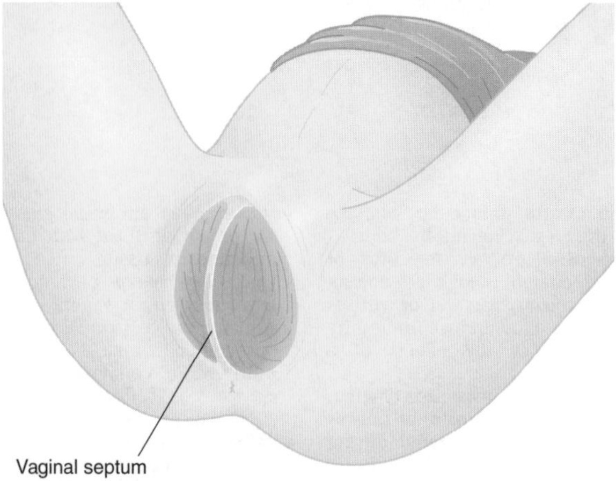

Vaginal septum

■ **Figure 144** Vaginal septum

vaginal speculum an instrument with two curved blades which can be inserted into the vagina and opened to allow for inspection of the walls and cervix.

vaginismus painful spasm of vaginal muscles.

vaginitis inflammation of the vagina. May be due to a fungus (*Candida albicans*) or to a flagellate protozoan (*Trichomonas vaginalis*), both of which cause a discharge and itching.

vagus the 10th cranial nerve which supplies and stimulates the lungs, heart, liver and stomach.

valgus a turning away from the mid-line of the body, e.g. *talipes valgus*.

validity the extent to which a test measurement or other device measures what it is intended to measure.

Valium® (diazepam) a moderately strong sedative widely used to reduce anxiety or treat convulsions.

Valsalva manoeuvre 1. a procedure originally created to aid the expulsion of ear wax whereby increased intrathoracic pressure is achieved by closing the glottis and forcing expiration. Has been used during the second stage of labour to cause pressure to increase in the abdomen thereby aiding the bearing-down efforts of the mother to deliver the baby. The practice is no longer encouraged as it is thought to contribute to fetal distress. 2. performed spontaneously by infants with respiratory distress syndrome to maintain a positive pressure in the thorax during expiration. A grunt results.

value 1. a belief about the worth of a given idea or behaviour. 2. a quantitative measurement of the activity or concentration of specific substances found in healthy tissue, blood, secretions, etc.

valve a natural or artificial structure present in a vessel which prevents backward flow of its contents.

vanillyl mandelic acid (VMA) a substance found normally in the urine. Increased levels indicate the presence of an adrenal tumour, a phaeochromocytoma.

variable a factor in an experiment or quantitative element that differs in values under changing conditions, e.g. the pulse at rest, during light exercise or during maximal exertion.

variance a numerical representation of the dispersion of data around the mean in a sample of results of research.

varicella a herpes-like viral infection. Causes chickenpox or shingles (herpes zoster).

varicose veins distended, bulging, dilated veins. The valves do not close efficiently allowing backflow of blood. In pregnancy the condition occurs under the influence of the hormone progesterone. Varicose veins may appear on the legs, vulva or round the rectum when they are called haemorrhoids.

variola smallpox.

varix an enlarged vein or a distended twisted lymphatic vessel.

vas a tube or vessel.

vas deferens the tube which carries spermatozoa from the testis to the male urethra.

vasa praevia the vessels from a velamentous insertion of the umbilical cord which run into the membranes, through to the placenta, and pass between the presenting part and the cervical opening. When the membranes rupture there is a risk that the vessels will rupture causing exsanguination, hypoxia, brain damage or death of the fetus.

vascular referring to blood vessels, usually small ones.

vascularity the amount of blood vessels in a given area or organ.

vasectomy dissection and excision of part of the vas deferens,

to prevent passage of spermatozoa (*see* Figure 145). The man is usually sterile after 3 months.

vasoconstrictor a drug, hormone or enzyme which causes narrowing of the lumen of blood vessels. It will affect blood pressure and the distribution of blood throughout the body.

vasodepressor an agent causing reduction of peripheral resistance to blood flow and resulting in lowering of blood pressure.

vasodilator a drug, hormone or enzyme which causes dilation of blood vessels by making smooth muscles of the vessels relax.

vasomotor referring to the nerves which control the contraction and relaxation of muscles of the blood vessels.

vasopressin a hormone produced by the posterior lobe of the pituitary gland. Acts on the kidneys to control water balance in the body. It has a marked antidiuretic property.

vasopressor usually a drug or hormone which stimulates contraction of the smooth muscle of vessels.

vault 1. a dome-shaped structure 2. the top part of the fetal skull which contains the cerebral hemispheres. Made up of two parietal bones, two frontal bones and the occiput. They are divided by membranes and fontanelles which allow overlapping (moulding) during birth (*see* Figure 146).

VDRL (Venereal Disease Research Laboratory) refers to a test which is done to detect syphilis.

vegan a person who does not eat or use any products of animal origin, i.e. meat, fish, dairy, eggs, leather, honey. Vegan women may also decline the routine use of pharmaceutical drugs derived from animal products (e.g. oxytocics, prostaglandins).

vegetarian a person who does not eat meat, fish or foods

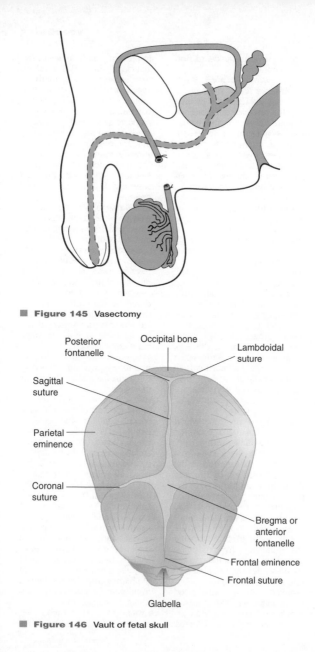

Figure 145 Vasectomy

Figure 146 Vault of fetal skull

Posterior fontanelle
Occipital bone
Lambdoidal suture
Sagittal suture
Parietal eminence
Coronal suture
Bregma or anterior fontanelle
Frontal eminence
Frontal suture
Glabella

made from the bodies of animals; a *lacto-ovo vegetarian* will eat dairy products and eggs; *complete vegetarian* is another term for vegan.

vein a vessel in the circulatory system which carries blood towards the heart.

vein of Galen the large cerebral vein that drains blood from the mid-brain.

velamentous veil-like.

velamentous insertion of the cord the cord is anchored in the membranes and the vessels divide before reaching the placenta.

vena cava two major veins running the length of the spine which return blood to the right upper chamber of the heart. The abdominal section can be compressed by the uterus when the pregnant woman lies on her back. Venous return to the heart will be inhibited causing pooling of blood in the abdominal cavity and reduced supply to the head. Dizziness, low blood pressure and fainting may result.

venepuncture perforation of a vein to obtain a specimen of blood for diagnostic testing.

venereal referring to sexual intercourse. *Venereal disease* is an infection transmitted from one person to another by sexual intercourse.

venesection opening of the vein to take blood or introduce drugs.

ventilation introduction of air into a room, or into the lungs by artificial means.

ventilator an apparatus used to force air mixed with oxygen into the lungs via an endotracheal tube using continuous or intermittent pressure.

Ventolin® (salbutamol) a drug inhaled or ingested which causes smooth muscles to relax; particularly useful for asthmatic patients or women in preterm labour.

ventouse extraction (vacuum extraction) the application of a cap to the fetal head when completion of the second stage of labour is delayed. The cap is attached to a machine which creates negative pressure. Traction can be applied which, with maternal efforts, may achieve delivery (*see* Figure 147).

ventricle a small cavity such as the lower chambers of the heart or the cavities in the brain filled with cerebrospinal fluid.

ventricular septal defect refers to a congenital abnormality of the heart. The wall dividing the right and left side of the heart is patent allowing blood from one side of the heart to flow to the other, bypassing the lungs.

ventrosuspension surgical procedure in which the abdomen is opened and the round ligaments supporting the uterus are shortened to change the uterus from being retroverted to anteverted.

venous stasis pooling or cessation in the flow of blood in a vein.

venous thrombosis formation of a blood clot in a vein which obstructs the flow through the vessel.

venule a tiny vein.

vernix caseosa a greasy substance secreted from the sebaceous glands. It covers the fetus in utero and falls off into the liquor at term.

verruca contagious skin condition caused by a virus.

version turning of the fetal position in utero. Cephalic version is turning to make the head present over the internal os. In external cephalic version (ECV) the fetus is manipulated through the abdominal wall until it is a cephalic presentation. Podalic version is turning the fetus to a breech position from an oblique lie or following delivery of a first

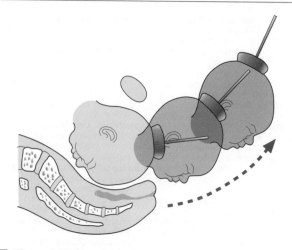

■ **Figure 147** Ventouse (vacuum) extraction

twin. In internal version the operator's hand is introduced into the uterus and a second twin is turned from a transverse lie in order to achieve a vaginal delivery.

vertebrae (SINGULAR vertebra) the irregular-shaped bones which form the spine and through the middle of which passes the spinal cord.

vertebral canal hollow channel in the vertebrae through which the spinal cord passes.

vertebral column the structure composed of 33 vertebrae resting one on top of another and divided by cartilage which encases the spinal cord, maintains rigidity and provides support to the upper body.

vertex the top of the fetal head bounded by the anterior and posterior fontanelles and the parietal eminences.

vesica the urinary bladder.

vesical referring to the urinary bladder or other fluid-filled sac.

vesical fistula an abnormal opening into the urinary bladder.

vesical sphincter the circular muscle which closes the bladder.

vesicle a blister or small sac usually containing fluid.

vesicouterine referring to the bladder and the uterus.

vesicovaginal referring to the bladder and vagina.

vesicular referring to or containing vesicles.

vestibule 1. entrance or passageway. 2. part of the vulva found between the labia minora.

vestige the remnants of a structure from fetal life.

viable capable of survival – as the fetus after 24 weeks' gestation.

viable fetus a fetus capable of survival, legally defined in the UK to be after 24 weeks' gestation, although in practice less rigid than this.

vicarious liability describes an agreement where an employer has responsibility for the actions carried out in the course of the employee's work.

villi fine, hair-like processes which project from skin or a mucous surface. Found in the lungs, intestines and placenta. *Chorionic villi* are processes around the trophoblast which grow into the maternal blood vessels.

viraemia viral infection of the blood.

viral referring to a virus.

viral infection occurring where a virus enters the body and attaches itself to a susceptible cell which absorbs the virus. The virus matures inside the cell using its own genetic information. It replicates itself in the parasitized cell. It will then appear outside the cell and seek new cells to parasitize.

viral load test a measurement of the amount of the human immunodeficiency virus in the blood.

virgin 1. a person who has never had sexual intercourse. 2. pure, uncontaminated.

virility referring to an adult male's capacity for procreation.

virus very small micro-organism which can only grow within another cell. Viruses can cross the placental barrier and cause congenital abnormalities in the first trimester.

viscera internal organs enclosed within a body cavity.

visceral cavity the abdominal cavity; the cavity of any organ, e.g. the stomach.

viscosity the resistance exhibited by a fluid as it flows over a surface.

viscous sticky, as thick mucous.

visual analogue scale (VAS) a method of quantifying feelings, e.g. pain. A line is drawn, one end representing no pain sensation the other severe pain. The patient is asked to plot the strength of his or her pain on the line. This may be used again to detect changes in the pain.

visual disturbance impairment of visual acuity. May be due to optic or cerebral oedema and may indicate the presence of pre-eclampsia or impending convulsion.

vital 1. very important. 2. relating to life.

vital signs temperature, pulse, respiratory rate, blood pressure, level of consciousness and responsiveness.

vital statistics record of births and deaths including causative factors in the population maintained by the Public Record Office.

vitamin essential food substances, minute amounts of which are necessary for health. Early classification divided them into groups from A to V. Deficiency of vitamins causes an array of conditions depending on which one is absent from the diet.

vitellin a protein containing lecithin found in egg yolk.

vitelline artery the vessels which circulate blood through the yolk sac to and from the embryo.

vitellus the yolk of an ovum.

viviparous classification of species that give birth to live offspring.

void to empty, usually the bladder.

voluntary an action or thought involving conscious decision.

volvulus twisting, usually of the intestines, causing an obstruction or strangulation.

vomiting forceful expulsion of the contents of the stomach; sign of a pathological process. *Projectile vomiting* is very forceful vomiting usually caused by pyloric stenosis. *Vomiting in the newborn* may be due to overfeeding, air or mucus in the stomach. *Vomiting in early pregnancy* is commonly called morning sickness; more usually the woman is nauseous due to the presence of unfamiliar hormones in quantity in the brain. *Severe vomiting in pregnancy* (hyperemesis gravidarum) can result in dehydration and electrolyte imbalance. *Vomiting in late pregnancy* may be due to impending eclampsia, gastroenteritis or the onset of labour.

vomitus the material which comes up from the stomach.

vulsellum a type of forceps.

vulva external part of the female genital organs.

vulvectomy cutting away of the vulva.

vulvitis inflammation of the vulva.

Ww

waiter's tip the position of the arm and hand being turned backwards, resulting from nerve damage and paralysis (Erb's palsy).

warfarin an oral anticoagulant drug which will cross the placental barrier. Only given between 16 and 36 weeks of pregnancy if clinically indicated.

wart a virus which invades the skin only causing a roughened elevation. *Genital warts* are found on the vulva, perineum and anal regions. They can be treated topically.

water birth birthing of the baby in water; more commonly used to describe the process of labouring in which warm water is used for relaxation and pain relief.

water intoxication excess water in the body to the extent that bodily functions are impaired.

waterborne protein, salt or micro-organism which moves about in water.

weaning changing the diet in an infant. There is a gradual change from milk to semisolid foods and then solid foods slowly over several months.

webbed connected by a fold of membrane or skin. These are more usually found between the toes and fingers.

wedge resection surgical removal of a wedge-shaped part of an organ, usually the ovary or cervix.

weight gain occurs in pregnancy, up to 12 kg.

well baby clinic a clinic where mothers of healthy babies can meet health care professionals and have their babies' development assessed and health monitored.

well-being individual sense of contentment with state of health.

well woman clinic a clinic concerned with screening apparently healthy women for detection of breast and cervical cancers and other conditions.

Wernicke's encephalopathy acute haemorrhagic encephalitis associated with severe hyperemesis gravidarum.

Wertheim's operation hysterectomy which is combined with removal of the ovaries, fallopian tubes, upper third of the vagina, perimetrium and clearance of pelvic lymph nodes. Used to treat cancer of the cervix.

wet nurse a woman who breastfeeds babies who are not her own.

Wharton's jelly the clear jelly-like substance surrounding the vessels of the umbilical cord.

whey the fluid part of milk which can be separated from the solid part, curds.

white blood cell (WBC) leukocytes found in the blood. Their function is to ingest foreign bodies and micro-organisms.

white matter white substance composed of myelinated nerve fibres, responsible for transmission of impulses up the spinal cord and across the brain.

whole blood donated blood is transfused without the removal of any components.

whooping cough (SYNONYM pertussis) a serious upper respiratory tract infection.

Wilson-Mikity syndrome a condition occurring in babies who have needed to be ventilated for a period of time; the lung tissue loses its elasticity.

withdrawal bleeding blood loss from the uterus occurring after the cessation of oestrogen and progesterone preparations, as happens with each course of oral contraceptive pills.

withdrawal method practice during intercourse in which the penis is removed from the vagina just before ejaculation.

withdrawal symptoms unpleasant possibly damaging symptoms which occur after cessation of a drug taken regularly for a long period of time.

womb uterus.

Woolwich shell a plastic domed appliance with a flat base containing a hole. Used to encourage retraction of flat nipples. The nipple is inserted into the hole and the appliance is worn inside the brassiere.

World Health Organization (WHO) special agency set up by the United Nations Council which is concerned with international health. It funds research and development, supports educational and local initiatives to improve environmental health. It initiated the Safe Motherhood campaign to improve maternal mortality in underdeveloped countries.

WHO International Code of Marketing of Breast Milk Substitutes a campaign started in conjunction with UNICEF to safeguard breast-feeding practice and regulate the advertising of breast milk substitutes by companies in developing countries. The code prevents direct advertising, free distribution of samples, special offers and discounts to mothers and professionals.

wound injury caused to the skin and underlying tissues by surgery, trauma or puncture.

wound healing process whereby integrity and function are restored to an injured part.

Wrigley's forceps obstetric forceps used to grip the fetal head. Traction is applied to effect delivery of the fetus when the second stage of labour is delayed. The head needs to be low in the pelvic cavity for a 'lift out'. They are also used during caesarean section or to control the aftercoming head in a medically managed breech delivery.

Xx

X chromosome one of two chromosomes that determine the gender of a cell. A cell with XX chromosomes will be female and a cell with XY chromosomes will be male.

xanthoderma skin with a yellow tinge, as in jaundice.

xenogenesis the changing of genes as they are passed down several generations to produce different traits.

xeroderma skin that is dry and rough.

xeromammogram a type of X-ray using metal plates instead of films for examining the breast.

X-linked refers to a disease acquired by recessive inheritance in which the defect is located on the X chromosome. The female will carry the condition without being affected and will pass it on to her male children who will be affected.

X-linked dominant inheritance passing on of a characteristic expressed whenever the gene is present on the X chromosome.

X-linked inheritance the passing on of traits on the X chromosome. These traits are maternally derived and will not be passed on by males to their sons but their daughters will be carriers and pass it to the next generation.

X-linked recessive inheritance a pattern of inheritance in which the females carry the trait and only the males show symptoms.

xiphoid process a small piece of cartilage at the end of the sternum against which the height of the uterine fundus is measured during pregnancy.

XO denotes a condition called Turner's syndrome in which only one chromosome (X) is present in each cell.

X-rays electromagnetic waves which can pass through many substances such as skin, muscle and paper but are absorbed by lead, bone and platinum. When a part of the skeleton is exposed to X-ray, images can be made of the bones and diseases including fractures detected.

X-ray pelvimetry radiological picture of the pelvis which can be measured to determine the dimensions. Rarely carried out in current practice.

Xylocaine® (lidocaine hydrochloride (lignocaine hydrochloride)) a drug given by injection which causes anaesthesia in the region in which it is injected.

XYY syndrome a condition in which the male has an extra Y chromosome making 47 in each cell instead of 46. The male is often aggressive, tall and displays antisocial behaviour.

Yy

Y chromosome the sex chromosome indicative of a male.

yaws a disease found in the tropics that resembles syphilis and is caused by *Treponema* but which is not a venereal disease. Tests for syphilis will be positive.

yeast a specific fungus which causes fruit juices and malt to ferment producing alcohol. Thrush is a yeast-type infection caused by *Candida albicans*.

yoga discipline of exercises focusing on posture, breathing and meditation to aid health and relaxation.

yolk sac a structure that develops in the inner cell mass and expands into a vesicle with a thick stalk that becomes the embryonic gut (*see* Figure 148). It supplies the nourishment for the developing embryo and disappears by the 7th week of gestation.

Yutopar® (ritodrine hydrochloride) a drug usually given intravenously which relaxes uterine muscles and is sometimes offered in an attempt to stop preterm labour.

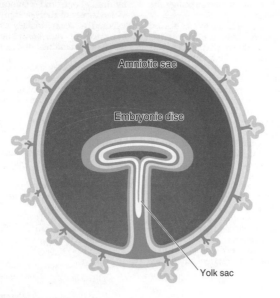

■ **Figure 148** Yolk sac

Zz

zero (0) the symbol meaning '0' – nought or nothing. It is also the point on a centigrade thermometer at which temperature measurement begins, water turns to ice or above which ice melts.

zinc an element essential in the diet for making enzymes. Deficiency can cause growth retardation in children, low sperm counts in men and slow wound healing.

zona fasciculata the middle part of the adrenal cortex which produces glucocorticoids and sex hormones.

zona pellucida the thick transparent secretory layer surrounding the ovum. A sperm's head contains an enzyme which digests this layer allowing penetration and fertilization.

Zovirax® (aciclovir) an antiviral agent used to treat viruses such as herpes simplex. It is applied locally but can be given intravenously.

zygogenesis joining to form a single unit; the formation of the zygote after fertilization.

zygonema a synaptic chromosome formation that occurs in the zygote in the meiotic prophase of gametogenesis.

zygote the fertilized ovum before it starts to divide.

zygote intrafallopian transfer (ZIFT) infertility treatment. Introduction of the fertilized ovum (prior to segmentation) into the fallopian tube.

Appendices

Appendix 1

Drugs and the law

The main acts governing the use of medicines are the Medicines Act 1968, the Misuse of Drugs Act 1971 and the Medicinal Products: Prescription by Nurses Act 1992.

The Medicines Act 1968 divides medicines into three groups:

- Prescription Only Medicines (POM)
- Pharmacy Only Medicines (P)
- General Sales List Medicines (GSL)

These distinctions do not apply to hospitals where it is accepted practice that all medicines are supplied only on prescription. Regulations that came into force on 9th August 2002[1] provide for **Patient Group Directions** to be drawn up to make provision for the sale or supply of a prescription only medicine in hospitals in accordance with the written direction of a doctor or dentist. These regulations enable specified health professionals, including midwives, to provide medicines without a doctor having first seen the patient, provided that a Patient Group Direction has been drawn up in accordance with the Regulations.

The midwife and controlled drugs

Registered midwives have specific statutory powers in relation to medicines and controlled drugs. A registered midwife who has notified the local supervising authority of her intention to practise may, as far as is necessary for the practice of her profession or employment as a midwife, possess and administer any Controlled Drug which the Medicines Act 1968 permits her to administer (Regulation 11 of the Misuse of Drugs Regulations 2001[2]). Supplies may only be made to her or possessed by her, on the authority of a midwife's supply order. This supply order must specify the name and occupation of the midwife, the purpose for which it is required and the total quantity to be obtained. The supply order must be signed by a doctor who is authorised by the local supervising authority for the region or area in which the Controlled Drug was, or is to be obtained or by the Supervisor of Midwives appointed by the local supervising authority for that area. The regulation defines a midwife's supply order as 'an order in writing specifying the name and occupation of the midwife obtaining the drug, the purpose for which it is required and the total quantity to be obtained'. By Statutory Instrument[3] the midwife can supply:

- All medicines that are not POM
- POM containing any of the following substances (but no other POM)
  - Chloral hydrate
  - Ergometrine maleate (only when contained in a medicinal product not for parenteral administration)
  - Pentazocine hydrochloride

- Phytomenadione[4]
- Triclofos sodium

The midwife can also administer parenterally in the course of professional practice POM containing any of the following substances[5]:

- Ergometrine maleate
- Lidocaine (lignocaine)*
- Lidocaine (lignocaine) hydrochloride*
- Naloxone hydrochloride
- Oxytocin, natural and synthetic
- Pentazocine lactate
- Pethidine hydrochloride
- Phytomenadione
- Promazine hydrochloride*

*Lidnocaine, lidnocaine hydrochloride and promazine hydrochloride may only be administered by a midwife whilst attending a woman in childbirth.

POM include most of the potent drugs in common use that can only be supplied and administered on the instructions of an appropriate practitioner (doctor, dentist or nurse prescriber). P refers to drugs supplied under the control and supervision of a registered pharmacist. GSL medicines are freely available over the counter through any retail outlet.

The Misuse of Drugs Act

The Misuse of Drugs (Supply to Addicts) Regulations 1997 amends the 1973 regulations. This act imposes controls on those drugs liable to produce dependence or cause harm if misused. It prohibits the possession, supply and manufacture of medicinal and other products, except where this has been made legal by the Misuse of Drugs Regulations 2001. The Misuse of Drugs Act categorises drugs into five separate schedules according to different levels of control. Midwives should be familiar with regulations governing Schedule 2 and Schedule 3 medicines. The substances cited in Schedule 2 of the Act are known as 'Controlled Drugs' and include:

- Amfetamine
- Cocaine
- Codeine injection
- Dexamfetamine
- Dextromoramide
- Diamorphine
- Dihydrocodeine injection
- Dipipanone
- Fentanyl
- Methadone
- Methylphenidate
- Morphine
- Pethidine
- Phenazocine

Schedule 3 includes medicines such as barbiturates, buprenorphine and temazepam, which are also controlled drugs.

It is no longer a requirement that doctors notify cases of drug misuse to the Home Office but they are now expected to report these to their local Drug Misuse Database (DMD), using a standard form. Phone numbers are set out in the British National Formulary (BNF).

Disposal of unwanted drug stocks

A midwife may surrender any stocks of Controlled Drugs in her possession which she no longer requires to the doctor as identified above (Reg.11) or any doctor, or pharmacist (Reg.6).

Documentation

The midwife must keep a Controlled Drug book in which she must record the following:

- The date
- The name and address of the person from whom the drug was obtained
- The amount obtained
- The form in which it was obtained
- The name and address of the patient to whom the drug was administered
- The amount administered
- The form in which it was administered

When the midwife receives the controlled drug from the pharmacist she must sign the Pharmacist's Controlled Drugs Register and the pharmacist must keep the midwife's supply order for two years.

Midwives rules[6]

Administration of medicines

The Midwives rules specify additional rules in relation to the supply and possession of medicines by midwives.

Rule 41 (as amended by the NMC in 2003) on the administration of medicines and other forms of pain relief sets out the following requirements:

- A practising midwife shall only administer medicines, including analgesics, in which she has been trained to use, dosage and methods of administration
- In a situation in which clinical trials involving new medicines including inhalational analgesics, or new apparatus, are taking place, a practising midwife may only participate under the direction of a registered medical practitioner.

Records

Under the rules revised by the NMC in 2003 Rule 42(5) now makes it a statutory duty for the self-employed midwife to transfer her official records to the local supervising authority immediately before she ceases to practice. This would include her documentation on medicines.

Inspection of premises and equipment

Rule 43 has been amended by the NMC so that the words in Rule 43(2) have been changed from 'shall use her best endeavours to permit inspection' to 'shall permit inspection of all institutional premises'. Under Rule 43(1) the midwife must give her supervisor of midwives, the local supervising authority and the NMC every reasonable facility to inspect her methods of practice, her records, her equipment and such part of her residence as may be used for professional purposes.

Midwives Code of Practice

The Midwives Code of Practice also provides guidance on the role of the midwife in relation to medicines. Unlike the Rules, these paragraphs are not part of the law of the country, but they provide guidance to registered midwives and failure to conform to the guidance could be used in evidence in professional conduct investigations and proceedings. The Code of Practice covers: Supply, possession and use of controlled drugs; Destruction and surrender of controlled drugs; Controlled drugs and home births; Prescription Only and other medicines used by midwives; the administration of homeopathic or herbal substances and the administration of controlled drugs.

Midwives may also be identified as the appropriate registered health professional to supply medicinal products to patients under a Patient Group Direction and would have to ensure that the statutory requirements for such authorisation have been complied (see above). Midwives may also be identified as extended formulary independent prescribers or supplementary prescribers (see above).

References

1. Prescription Only Medicines (Human Use) Amendment Order 2000 SI 2000 No 1917
2. Misuse of Drugs Regulations SI 2001 No 3998 amending and re-enacting the Misuse of Drugs Regulations SI 1985 2066
3. Statutory Instrument 1997 No 1830
4. Statutory Instrument 1998 No 2081
5. Statutory Instrument 1997 No 1830
6. UKCC Midwives Rules and Code of Practice 1998 revised by the Nursing and Midwifery Council 2003.

Appendix 2

Tests

Aminocentesis

To assess fetal maturity and diagnose fetal abnormalities.

Bicarbonate in whole arterial blood

Detects acidosis and alkalosis. Normal range 18–23 mmol/l.

Bilirubin

Indicator of the extent of haemoglobin destruction. Levels may be elevated in some medical conditions. Liver disease, obstructive jaundice, haemolytic anaemia and pulmonary infarct. Normal range 2–17 μmol/l.

Chorionic gonadotrophin

Assessment of level in EMU to diagnose pregnancy.

Agglutination inhibition assay can be positive of pregnancy 8–14 days after missed period.

Monoclonal antibody test – positive if pregnancy 14–18 days following conception.

Chorionic villus sampling

Enables chromosomal analysis. Sample of CV obtained between 9 and 11 weeks gestation.

Cordocentesis

Chromosomal and haemoglobinopathies to be diagnosed in pregnancy.

Needling of umbilical cord and obtaining of fetal blood sample at around 18–19 weeks of pregnancy.

Enzyme-linked immunosorbent assay (ELISA)

Diagnosis of pregnancy.

Measurement of HCG in urine may give a positive pregnancy test 8–10 days following fertilization.

False negative is high if test is done too early or on excessively dilute urine.

Oral GTT

Diagnosis of impaired glucose tolerance of diabetes.

Fast for 10–16 hours
Glucose iode of 75 g over 5 mm
Serum glucose levels measured

Range at end of fast   3.9–5.8 mmol/l
                      30 mins 6.1–9.4 mmol/l
                      60 mins 6.7–9.4 mmol/l
                      90 mins 5.6–7.8 mmol/l
                   120 mins 3.9–6.7 mmol/l

Glycated (Glycosylated) Hb

Assess level of diabetic control and is an indicator of blood glucose level concentration over the previous 4–8 weeks.

Normal range in insulin dependent diabetics 7–9 per cent.

Hepatitis A antigens and hepatitis B surface antigen. Not normally present, thus when found is indicative of infection.

Hep A Anti-HAV IgG appears about 4/52 after infection and persists indefinitely.

HB indicative of viral infection.

HIV antibodies

Not normally present in blood. Detection of antibodies can be as early as 4 weeks but may take 4/12 to appear following infection and persists indefinitely.

ELISA used for assessment.

LFT

Chemical detectors
    Bilirubin
    Albumin
    Alkaline phosphatase (a bile enzyme)
    Amino transferase for transaminase (produced following liver-cell damage)
    Prothrombin time (a blood test) but indicator of the activity of vitamin K which is normally synthesized by the liver.

Prothrombin test (PT)

Measures amt of PT in blood function and integrity of clotting function. Normal range 10–14 seconds.

Serum amylase

To determine liver and pancreatic function. Normal range 25–125 U/l (units per litre).

Appendix 3

The Apgar scoring system
(to assess neonatal condition at birth)

	Score		
Sign	0	1	2
Heart rate	Absent	Slow – below 100	Fast – above 100
Respiratory effort	Absent	Slow, irregular	Good, crying
Muscle tone	Limp	Some flexion of the extremities	Active
Reflex irritability	No response	Grimace	Crying, cough
Colour	Blue, pale	Body pink, extremities blue	Completely pink

Appendix 4

Bart's test

Interpretation of risk factors

Maternal age	Risk of screen-positive result for Down's syndrome
Below 25	1:45
25–29	1:30
30–34	1:15
35–39	1:5
40–44	1:2
Over 45	More than 1:2

Appendix 5

Modified Bishop's scoring system (to assess favourability of cervix for induction of labour)

Assessment features	0	1	2	3
Dilatation of the cervix (cm)	0	1–2	3–4	5–6
Consistency of the cervix	Firm	Medium	Soft	–
Length of cervical canal (cm)	>2	1–2	0.5–1	<0.5
Position of cervix	Posterior	Mid	Anterior	–
Station of presenting part related to ischial spines	–3	–2	–3	+1, +2

When the total score is greater than eight the cervix is said to be favourable (Royal College of Obstetricians and Gynaecologists (2001) Induction of labour. Evidence-based Clinical Guideline No. 9. London, RCOG Press)

Appendix 6

The Dubowitz score (to assess neonatal maturity)

External (superficial) Criteria

External sign	0	1
OEDEMA	Obvious oedema hands and feet: pitting over tibia	No obvious oedema hands and feet: pitting over tibia
SKIN TEXTURE	Very thin, gelatinous	Thin and smooth
SKIN COLOUR (infant not crying)	Dark red	Uniformly pink
SKIN OPACITY (trunk)	Numerous veins and venules clearly seen, especially over abdomen	Veins and tributaries seen
LANUGO (over back)	No lanugo	Abundant; long and thick over whole back
PLANTAR CREASES	No skin creases	Faint red marks over anterior half of sole
NIPPLE FORMATION	Nipple barely visible; no areola	Nipple well defined; areola smooth and flat diameter <0.75 cm
BREAST SIZE	No breast tissue palpable	Breast tissue on one or both sides <0.5 cm diameter
EAR FORM	Pinna flat and shapeless, little or no incurving edge	Incurving of part of edge of pinna
EAR FIRMNESS	Pinna soft, easily folded, no recoil	Pinna soft, easily folded, slow recoil
GENITALIA MALE	Neither testis in scrotum	At least one testis high in scrotum
FEMALE (with hips half abducted)	Labia majora widely separated, labia minora protruding	Labia majora almost cover labia minora

(Adapted from Farr et al., *Develop. Med. Child Neurol.* (1966) **8**, 507)

Score		
2	**3**	**4**
No oedema		
Smooth: medium thickness. Rash or superficial peeling	Slight thickening. Superficial cracking and peeling esp. hand and feet	Thick and parchment-like; superficial or deep cracking
Pale pink: variable over body	Pale. Only pink over ears, lips, palms or soles	
A few large vessels clearly seen over abdomen	A few large vessels seen indistinctly over abdomen	No blood vessels seen
Hair thinning especially over lower back	Small amount of lanugo and bald areas	At least half of back devoid of lanugo
Definite red marks over more than anterior half; indentations over less than anterior third	Indentations over more than anterior third	Definite deep indentations over more than anterior third
Areola stippled, edge not raised; diameter <0.75 cm	Areola stippled, edge raised diameter >0.75 cm	
Breast tissue both sides; one or both 0.5–1.0 cm	Breast tissue both sides; one or both >1 cm	
Partial incurving whole of upper pinna	Well-defined incurving whole of upper pinna	
Cartilage to edge of pinna, but soft in places, ready recoil	Pinna firm, cartilage to edge, instant recoil	
At least one testis right down		
Labia majora completely cover labia minora		

Appendix 7

Newborn life support

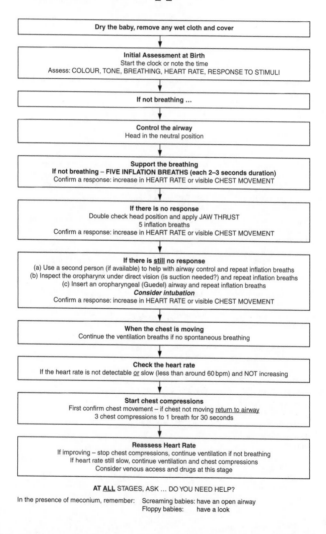

| Dry the baby, remove any wet cloth and cover |

Initial Assessment at Birth
Start the clock or note the time
Assess: COLOUR, TONE, BREATHING, HEART RATE, RESPONSE TO STIMULI

If not breathing ...

Control the airway
Head in the neutral position

Support the breathing
If not breathing – FIVE INFLATION BREATHS (each 2–3 seconds duration)
Confirm a response: increase in HEART RATE or visible CHEST MOVEMENT

If there is no response
Double check head position and apply JAW THRUST
5 inflation breaths
Confirm a response: increase in HEART RATE or visible CHEST MOVEMENT

If there is still no response
(a) Use a second person (if available) to help with airway control and repeat inflation breaths
(b) Inspect the oropharynx under direct vision (is suction needed?) and repeat inflation breaths
(c) Insert an oropharyngeal (Guedel) airway and repeat inflation breaths
Consider intubation
Confirm a response: increase in HEART RATE or visible CHEST MOVEMENT

When the chest is moving
Continue the ventilation breaths if no spontaneous breathing

Check the heart rate
If the heart rate is not detectable or slow (less than around 60 bpm) and NOT increasing

Start chest compressions
First confirm chest movement – if chest not moving return to airway
3 chest compressions to 1 breath for 30 seconds

Reassess Heart Rate
If improving – stop chest compressions, continue ventilation if not breathing
If heart rate still slow, continue ventilation and chest compressions
Consider venous access and drugs at this stage

AT **ALL** STAGES, ASK ... DO YOU NEED HELP?

In the presence of meconium, remember: Screaming babies: have an open airway
Floppy babies: have a look

Appendix 8

Management of cardiac arrest

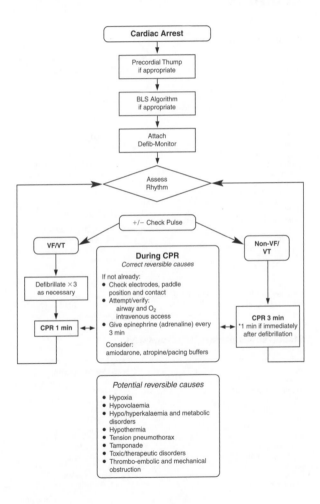

Cardiac Arrest

Precordial Thump
if appropriate

BLS Algorithm
if appropriate

Attach
Defib-Monitor

Assess
Rhythm

+/– Check Pulse

VF/VT

Non-VF/
VT

Defibrillate ×3
as necessary

CPR 1 min

CPR 3 min
*1 min if immediately
after defibrillation

During CPR
Correct reversible causes

If not already:
- Check electrodes, paddle
  position and contact
- Attempt/verify:
  airway and O$_2$
  intravenous access
- Give epinephrine (adrenaline) every
  3 min

Consider:
amiodarone, atropine/pacing buffers

Potential reversible causes
- Hypoxia
- Hypovolaemia
- Hypo/hyperkalaemia and metabolic
  disorders
- Hypothermia
- Tension pneumothorax
- Tamponade
- Toxic/therapeutic disorders
- Thrombo-embolic and mechanical
  obstruction

Appendix 9

Normal blood/urine values in adults

Blood (haematology)

Test	Reference range
Activated partial thromboplastin time (APTT)	30–40 s
Bleeding time (Ivy)	2–8 min
Erythrocyte sedimentation rate (ESR)	
Adult women	3–15 mm/h
Adult men	1–10 mm/h
Fibrinogen	1.5–4.0 g/L
Folate (serum)	4–18 µg/L
Haemoglobin	
Women	115–165 g/L (11.5–16.5 g/dL)
Men	130–180 g/L (13–18 g/dL)
Haptoglobins	0.3–2.0 g/L
Mean cell haemoglobin (MCH)	27–32 pg
Mean cell haemoglobin concentration (MCHC)	30–35 g/dL
Mean cell volume (MCV)	78–95 fl
Packed cell volume (PCV or haematocrit)	
Women	0.35–0.47 (35–47%)
Men	0.4–0.54 (40–54%)
Platelets (thrombocytes)	$150–400 \times 10^9$/L
Prothrombin time	12–16 s
Red cells (erythrocytes)	
Women	$3.8–5.3 \times 10^{12}$/L
Men	$4.5–6.5 \times 10^{12}$/L
Reticulocytes (newly formed red cells in adults)	$25–85 \times 10^9$/L
White cells total (leucocytes)	$4.0–11.0 \times 10^9$/L

Blood-venous plasma (biochemistry)

Test	Reference range
Alanine aminotransferase (ALT)	10–40 U/L
Albumin	36–47 g/L
Alkaline phosphatase	40–125 U/L
Amylase	90–300 U/L
Aspartate aminotransferase (AST)	10–35 U/L
Bicarbonate (arterial)	22–28 mmol/L
Bilirubin (total)	2–17 µmol/L
Caeruloplasmin	150–600 mg/L
Calcium	2.1–2.6 mmol/L
Chloride	95–105 mmol/L
Cholesterol (total)	ideally below 5.2 mmol/L

(Continued)

Blood-venous plasma (biochemistry) (continued)

Test	Reference range
HDL-Cholesterol	
Women	0.6–1.9 mmol/L
Men	0.5–1.6 mmol/L
$PaCO_2$ (arterial)	4.4–6.1 kPa
Copper	13–24 μmol/L
Cortisol (at 08.00 h)	160–565 nmol/L
Creatine kinase (total)	
Women	30–150 U/L
Men	30–200 U/L
Creatinine	55–150 μmol/L
Gamma-glutamyl-transferase (γGT)	
Women	5–35 U/L
Men	10–55 U/L
Globulins	24–37 kg/L
Glucose (venous blood, fasting)	3.6–5.8 mmol/L
Glycosylated haemoglobin (HbA_1)	4–6%
Hydrogen ion concentration (arterial)	35–44 nmol/L
Iron	
Women	10–28 μmol/L
Men	14–32 μmol/L
Iron-binding capacity total (TIBC)	45–70 μmol/L
Lactate (arterial)	0.3–1.4 mmol/L
Lactate dehydrogenase (total)	230–460 U/L
Lead (adults, whole blood)	<1.7 μmol/L
Magnesium	0.7–1.0 mmol/L
Osmolality	275–290 mmol/kg
PaO_2 (arterial)	12–15 kPa
Oxygen saturation (arterial)	>97%
pH	7.36–7.42
Phosphate (fasting)	0.8–1.4 mmol/L
Potassium (serum)	3.6–5.0 mmol/L
Protein (total)	60–80 g/L
Sodium	136–145 mmol/L
Transferrin	2–4 g/L
Triglycerides (fasting)	0.6–1.8 mmol/L
Urate	
Women	0.12–0.36 mmol/L
Men	0.12–0.42 mmol/L
Urea	2.5–6.5 mmol/L
Uric acid	
Women	0.09–0.36 mmol/L
Men	0.1–0.45 mmol/L
Vitamin A	0.7–3.5 μmol/L
Vitamin C	23–57 μmol/L
Zinc	11–22 μmol/L

Appendices

Cerebrospinal fluid

Test	Reference range
Cells	0–5 mm^3
Chloride	120–170 mmol/L
Glucose	2.5–4.0 mmol/L
Pressure (adult)	50–180 mm/H$_2$O
Protein	100–400 mg/L

Urine

Test	Reference range
Albumin/creatinine ratio	<3.5 mg albumin/mmol creatinine
Calcium (diet dependent)	<12 mmol/24 h (normal diet)
Copper	0.2–0.6 μmol/24 h
Cortisol	9–50 μmol/24 h
Creatinine	9–17 mmol/24 h
5-Hydroxyindole-3-acetic acid (5HIAA)	10–45 μmol/24 h
Magnesium	3.3–5.0 mmol/24 h
Oxalate	
Women	40–320 mmol/24 h
Men	80–490 mmol/24 h
pH	4–8
Phosphate	15–50 mmol/24 h
Porphyrins (total)	90–370 nmol/24 h
Potassium (depends on intake)	25–100 mmol/24 h
Protein (total)	no more than 0.3 g/L
Sodium (depends on intake)	100–200 mmol/24 h
Urea	170–500 mmol/24 h

Faeces

Test	Reference range
Fat content (daily output on normal diet)	<7 g/24 h
Fat (as stearic acid)	11–18 mmol/24 h

Appendix 10

Conversion charts

**Measurements, equivalents and conversions
(SI or metric and imperial)**

Length

1 kilometre (km)	= 1000 metres (m)
1 metre (m)	= 100 centimetres (cm) or 1000 millimetres (mm)
1 centimetre (cm)	= 10 millimetres (mm)
1 millimetre (mm)	= 1000 micrometres (μm)
1 micrometre (μm)	= 1000 nanometres (nm)

Conversions

1 metre (m)	= 39.370 inches (in)
1 centimetre (cm)	= 0.3937 inches (in)
30.48 centimetres (cm)	= 1 foot (ft)
2.54 centimetres (cm)	= 1 inch (in)

Volume

1 litre (L)	= 1000 millilitres (mL)
1 millilitre (mL)	= 1000 microlitres (μL)

NB The millilitre (mL) and the cubic centimetre (cm³) are usually treated as being the same.

Conversions

1 litre (L)	= 1.76 pints (pt)
568.25 millilitres (mL)	= 1 pint (pt)
28.4 millilitres (mL)	= 1 fluid ounce (fl oz)

Weight or mass

1 kilogram (kg)	= 1000 grams (g)
1 gram (g)	= 1000 milligrams (mg)
1 milligram (mg)	= 1000 micrograms (μg)
1 microgram (μg)	= 1000 nanograms (ng)

NB To avoid any confusion with milligram (mg) the word microgram (μg) should be written in full on prescriptions.

Conversions

1 kilogram (kg)	= 2.204 pounds (lb)
1 gram (g)	= 0.0353 ounce (oz)
453.59 grams (g)	= 1 pound (lb)
28.34 grams (g)	= 1 ounce (oz)

Temperature conversions

To convert Celsius to Fahrenheit:
multiply by 9, divide by 5, and add 32 to the result,
e.g. 36°C to Fahrenheit:
$36 \times 9 = 324 \div 5 = 64.8 + 32 = 96.8°F$
therefore 36°C = 96.8°F

To convert Fahrenheit to Celsius:
subtract 32, multiply by 5, and divide by 9,
e.g. 104°F to Celsius:
$104 - 32 = 72 \times 5 = 360 \div 9 = 40°C$
therefore 104°F = 40°C

Appendix 11

SI units

Base units

Quantity	Base unit and symbol
Length	metre (m)
Mass	kilogram (kg)
Time	second (s)
Amount of substance	mole (mol)
Electric current	ampere (A)
Thermodynamic temperature	kelvin (K)
Luminous intensity	candela (cd)

Quantity	Derived unit and symbol
Work, energy, quantity of heat	joule (J)
Pressure	pascal (Pa)
Force	newton (N)
Frequency	hertz (Hz)
Power	watt (W)
Electrical potential, electromotive force, potential difference	volt (v)
Absorbed dose of radiation	gray (Gy)
Radioactivity	becquerel (Bq)
Dose equivalent	sievert (Sv)

Multiplication factor	Prefix	Symbol
10^{12}	tera	T
10^{9}	giga	G
10^{6}	mega	M
10^{3}	kilo	k
10^{2}	hecto	h
10^{1}	deca	da
10^{-1}	deci	d
10^{-2}	centi	c
10^{-3}	milli	m
10^{-6}	micro	μ
10^{-9}	nano	n
10^{-12}	pico	p
10^{-15}	femto	f
10^{-18}	atto	a

Appendix 12

The signs and progress of labour

Sara Wickham

Each woman's labour is a unique and individual journey. The same woman may, over the course of her childbearing experiences, have very different labours, and no two women will experience their labours the same way. For this reason, any midwife's understanding of the signs and progress of labour needs to be fluid, flexible and adaptable to the unique situation of each individual woman. While there are general themes that can be drawn into a discussion of the journey of labour, there should never be an assumption that any particular sign or rate of progress can be applied to all women.

In recent years, established labour has been divided into a number of relatively arbitrary stages, including the latent phase and the established phase, to differentiate early labour from the 'hard' labour which demands the woman's full attention. Practitioners then talk about the first, second, third and sometimes fourth stages of labour; denoting, respectively, the dilation of the cervix, the pushing stage and birth of the baby, the birth of the placenta and membranes and the recovery of the woman and establishment of breastfeeding. In reality, the labouring woman does not recognise these distinctions in a journey which flows from one moment to the next.

Signs of labour

Signs of early labour (also known as the latent phase of labour) include **nesting**, where the woman may experience a desire to clean or re-organise her living space; **backache, low abdominal pain or cramping** and/or a **show** – the release of the protective plug of mucus from the cervix as **effacement** and **dilation** begin. The woman may notice slight changes in her **baby's movement or behaviour** and may experience several days of 'early' labour before feeling her **contractions** begin or increase in intensity. She may experience the **spontaneous rupturing of her membranes** at any point from before labour begins until the baby's birth is imminent.

Early labour can be a time of stress to women; definitions such as 'false' labour are not generally helpful to a woman who is unable to sleep well or who is experiencing very uncomfortable contractions or backache. Yet it may sometimes be appropriate to gently remind women that harder work may lie ahead and that, as far as possible, they should try to rest and conserve their energy for the time when labour progresses further.

When talking to a woman who is in early labour, the midwife needs to help the woman make a decision about where she feels she is in her labour and whether she needs a midwife to go to her home, or, if she is planning a hospital or birth centre birth, to make plans to travel there. This decision needs to be finely balanced; the woman may be seeking reassurance that her labour is normal, and therefore want to see a midwife or go to hospital, yet if she goes into a hospital at an early stage her labour may not continue to progress as it might have in her own environment.

The progress of labour

At some point, labour is deemed to have become 'established'. This is said to occur when the woman's cervix has reached four centimetres dilation and her contractions are strong and regular. Yet some women may reach four centimetres dilation a week or two before labour begins, and others will be in strong labour well before their cervix is dilated to four centimetres.

As labour progresses, contractions become stronger and the cervix effaces and then dilates, while the baby moves down the birth canal. The strength and frequency of contractions may change over the course of labour, as do the sensations experienced by the labouring woman. Around the time the cervix has become fully dilated, the woman may experience an urge to push, or bear down, and, if encouraged to listen to her body, will follow this urge and push her baby out.

In a physiological labour (and third stage), after the baby is born, a few minutes usually go by before the woman again feels uterine contractions. Placental separation may be accompanied by a lengthening of the umbilical cord (as seen at the entrance to the vagina) and a small gush of blood. Within a few minutes, the woman may again feel an urge to push, or say that she feels something in her vagina; these signs usually occur just before the birth of the placenta. Some women spontaneously push their placentas out in response to these sensations, some women find their placenta is born with little effort on their part, and a few women may need some encouragement to push out their placenta.

Applying limits to labour

With the advent of medicalised birth, clinicians began to monitor and record the time taken for the various stages of labour to occur; a practice which, in theory, can be useful in order to establish when labour is progressing within normal limits and when it has become obstructed. In reality, the time limits applied to labour are often rigid and unreasonable, especially where women are giving birth in hospital environments which may not be conducive to their relaxation and physiological progress in labour. Frequently, women's labours fall outside the specified time limits and are then subject to medical intervention to speed up labour or expedite the birth of the baby and/or placenta.

The partogram, as a tool to monitor the progress of labour, should be seen in context; while it may be intended as a useful instrument to ensure that labour remains within normal limits, the application of this in all labouring women will mean that some of these women become subject to potentially unnecessary intervention because the progress of their labours fall outside of the norms set by local policies.

Assessing a woman's progress in labour

A woman's progress in labour can be assessed in a number of ways, either individually or in combination; the list that follows is by no means exhaustive.

Way of assessing progress	Examples
Sensations felt by the woman	The pattern of contractions varies during labour; descent of the fetal head causes the urge to push; crowning causes a burning sensation.
Observing the woman's behaviour	Women can talk more in early labour than late labour; women become more tired and irritable at the transition between the first and second stages.
The woman's prior experience	The woman may feel a sensation she experienced during the birth of a previous baby, such as the placenta entering the vagina.
Variations in contractions	Contractions tend to become closer together as first stage progresses; there may be a lull at the beginning of the second stage.
The purple line	A line can be seen extending up the buttock crease of women in labour as the cervix dilates (see Hobbs (1998) for more information).
Changing position of the fetal heart	The position on the woman's abdomen at which the fetal heart can be heard most clearly will become lower as labour progresses.
Changes in the fetal heart pattern	It is normal for the fetal heart to be heard to decelerate (and recover) as the woman pushes in second stage; this happens as the baby comes through the pelvis.
Abdominal examination	On palpation, the baby can be felt to move downwards over the course of the woman's labour, although women in labour do not always want to be palpated!
Vaginal examination	Changes in the dilation of the cervix and station of the head can be felt on vaginal examination if the woman is happy for you to do this (see Warren 1999).

References

Hobbs, L (1998) Assessing cervical dilation without VEs: watching the purple line. The Practising Midwife, 1(11), 34.
Warren, C (1999) Why should I do vaginal examinations? The Practising Midwife, 2(6), 12.

Both of these articles are republished in:
Wickham, S (Ed) (2003) Midwifery Best Practice. Books for Midwives' Press, Oxford.

Appendix 13

Fetal position and descent of the head

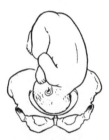

Fig A13.1 Left occipitoanterior

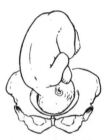

Fig A13.2 Right occipitoanterior

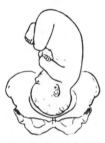

Fig A13.3 Left occipitolateral

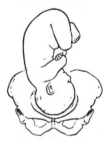

Fig A13.4 Right occipitolateral

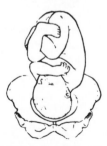

Fig A13.5 Left occipitoposterior

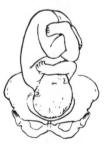

Fig A13.6 Right occipitoposterior

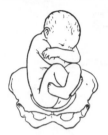

Fig A13.7 Right sacroposterior **Fig A13.8** Left sacroposterior

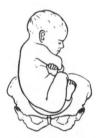
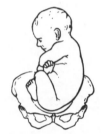

Fig A13.9 Right sacrolateral **Fig A13.10** Left sacrolateral

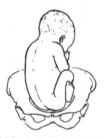
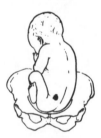

Fig A13.11 Right sacroanterior **Fig A13.12** Left sacroanterior

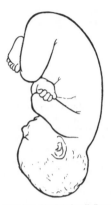

Fig A13.13 Vertex (well-flexed head)

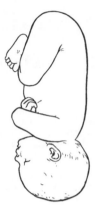

Fig A13.14 Vertex (deflexed head)

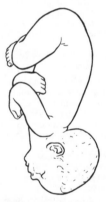

Fig A13.15 Brow (partially extended head)

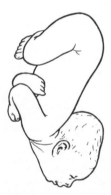

Fig A13.16 Face (fully extended head)

Appendix 14

Anti-D and choice

Anti-D is a pharmaceutical drug offered to rhesus negative women who have given birth to a rhesus positive baby, and in some areas to rhesus negative women during pregnancy. Anti-D is one of the medical world's success stories; a product which was developed in response to the problem of rhesus disease in the newborn. Since its discovery, thousands of babies have been saved from this disease, and its effects. Few midwives question the validity of anti-D; rather, they feel grateful for its existence. However, more and more women are declining anti-D, for a variety of reasons.

Rhesus disease can develop where a rhesus negative woman becomes *isoimmunised* – rhesus positive blood has entered her bloodstream and her body has (quite naturally) developed antibodies to fight off the foreign blood proteins. If an isoimmunised woman becomes pregnant with a rhesus positive baby, her antibodies can cross the placenta where they may haemolyse the baby's rhesus positive blood and cause the unborn baby to have the potentially serious *rhesus disease*.

There are a number of key issues in this area which midwives should be aware of and be able to discuss with women.

- Clinical trials carried out to test the effectiveness of anti-D showed that it was very effective in preventing isoimmunisation but that this does not automatically happen to all women; around 1 in 10 rhesus negative women who have given birth to a rhesus positive baby in a medicalised setting will become isoimmunised without anti-D. Some of the trials carried out in this area had serious methodological flaws.
- On the other hand, on a population level, appropriate use of anti-D reduces the risk of rhesus disease to a negligible level. Those midwives who have seen babies with severe rhesus disease are quick to detail the horrific effects this can have.
- The known and documented side effects of anti-D include local inflammation, "malaise, chills, fever and, rarely, anaphylaxis."[1] Some women have reported suffering an intensely irritating rash covering all, or most, of their body following the administration of anti-D, although this does not appear to have been documented in the midwifery or medical literature.
- Anti-D is a blood product which, despite being subject to purification processes, cannot be guaranteed completely safe. The risk of this is compounded by the fact that blood is pooled to make anti-D, and blood from one initial donor may end up in several hundred

*Unless otherwise stated, data in this appendix have been gathered from *Wickham S (2001) Anti-D in Midwifery: Panacea or Paradox? Books for Midwives Press, Oxford.*

doses of the end product. Several years ago, nearly 3000 women contracted hepatitis C from anti-D given in Ireland,[2] and there has been debate about whether HIV could also be transmitted through anti-D.[3]

- Some pharmaceutical companies use a mercury-based preservative, and the potential hazards of this are also making some women question whether they should accept anti-D.
- There is no evidence about the long-term effects of anti-D on women or unborn babies where this substance is given during pregnancy.
- There are a number of tests which can enable women to gather more information about their particular situation, including direct and indirect Coombes, Kleihauer and paternal blood typing.
- Currently, there appear to be no alternative products available. Although there are herbal or similar equivalents for most medical treatments, and homeopathic alternatives to issues such as vaccination, there does not seem yet to be a 'natural alternative' to anti-D.

Midwives, then, need to ensure that they are up-to-date with current evidence surrounding this issue and able to offer information to women in order to enable them to make informed choices about such issues.

References

1. British Medical Association and the Royal Pharmaceutical Society of Great Britain (1998) *British National Formulary* (Number 36). BMA/The Pharmaceutical Press, London.
2. Meisel H, Reip A, Faltus B (1995) Transmission of hepatitis C virus to children and husbands by women infected with contaminated anti-D immunoglobulin. *Lancet*, Vol. 345, No. 8959, 13 May 1995, pp 1209–1211.
3. Dumasia A, Kulkarni S, Joshi SH (1989) Women receiving anti-Rho(D) immunoglobulin containing HIV antibodies (correspondence). *Lancet*, Vol II, No. 8660, 19 August 1989, p 459.

Appendix 15

CV building blocks

Contact information

Your full name, address and postcode, phone numbers (home and mobile) and e-mail address.

Personal profile (optional)

A focused summary of your offer.

Designed to grab the reader's attention and highlight what is to come.

Summarises what you have to offer in a way that links to the employer's needs.

Key skills and competencies (optional)

A focused summary of your key skills.

Matches the employer's needs in terms of job and organisation.

Highlights transferable skills and competencies, which can be useful if you're changing direction.

Work experience

Start with your most recent position and work backwards.

Employers are usually interested in your most recent jobs, so concentrate on your last two positions – although you might occasionally want to highlight earlier roles.

Treat a promotion like a separate position.

Give the job title, when you started and left the job, the name of the company and a brief description of what they do.

List any of your main responsibilities, achievements, duties and skills that relate to the new position.

Describe the scope of your job and level of responsibility rather than giving task lists or a job description.

Highlight your achievements and successes such as increased sales, meeting deadlines, cost savings. You can do this job by job or in a separate section early on in the CV. Back them up with numerical evidence ('Increased sales by £50,000 over 6 months').

If you've had a lot of different roles or a long career, summarise just the key points about earlier roles under a subheading such as 'Previous employers' or 'Earlier career' or 'Background'.

Explain any significant gaps such as career breaks or unemployment.

Qualifications, education, training and development

Usually these come near the end, but if particular qualifications are essential for the job and make you more marketable (for example in technical and IT roles), put them on the first page after your profile or key skills.

Start with the most recent ones as they are of most value.

Give relevant professional qualifications and academic ones, but don't include 'bought' memberships.

List degrees or any executive programmes you have attended and give the subject, awarding body and year so they can be checked.

Summarise your school achievements briefly (e.g. 3 A-levels and 8 GCSEs). Only list the subjects if they are particularly relevant to your future role or if you haven't got a degree.

Add any relevant skills such as languages, technology, vocational or on the job training.

Include any relevant training or skills acquired while unemployed, on sabbatical or doing part-time or voluntary work.

Personal information

Date of birth (rather than age).

Single or married (if divorced put single, if separated put married – never include any kind of 'failure' on a CV).

Nationality – only if you're applying for jobs abroad.

Apart from those basics, anything else you add here must add value to your offer. Charitable activities may match an organisation's public commitment to working in the community.

Don't put driving experience if it's not relevant.

References and client endorsements

Referees are no longer included on CVs – although client references could support your CV in a portfolio.

But you can include client endorsements and recommendations in the achievements section of your CV – for example 'Given a special award by Anyco for contribution to ABC project'.

Cultural differences

CVs in Europe usually include detailed descriptions of schooling and higher education.

You might be asked to enclose a photo, particularly in Germany.

Photographs

You might also be asked for photos if you are applying to sectors that select partly on appearance (airlines, retail, customer facing activities or in companies where personal appearance is seen as part of 'living the brand').

If you need a photo, make sure it's a good quality one – not from a photo booth.

Interviewers often take digital photos at interviews to help them remember people.

Appendix 16

Useful addresses

Adoption UK Newborn

Manor Farm
Appletree Road
Chipping Warden
Banbury
Oxfordshire
OX17 1LH
Helpline: 0870 7700 450
Fax: 01295 660123
Website: www.adoptionuk.org.uk
Email: admin@adoptionuk.org.uk

Association for Postnatal Illness

25 Jordan Place
Fulham
London
SW6 1BE

Association for Spina Bifida and Hydrocephalus

ASBAH House
42 Park Road
Peterborough
PE1 2UQ
Tel: 01733 555988
Fax: 01733 555985
Website: www.asbeh.org
Email: postmaster@asbah.org

Audit Commission

1 Vincent Square
London
SW1P 2PN
Tel: 020 7828 1212
Website: www.auditcommission.gov.uk

Brook Advisory Centres

165 Grey's Inn Road
London
WC1X 8UD
Tel: 0171 713 9000
Website: www.brook.org.uk

Cleft-lip and Palate Association (CLAPA)

3rd Floor 235–237 Finchley Road
London
NW3 6LS
Tel: 020 7431 0033
Fax: 020 7431 8811
Website: www.clapa.com
Email: info@clapa.com

Commission for Health Improvement (CHI)

3rd Floor
Hannibal House
Elephant and Castle
London
SE1 6UD
Tel: 020 7277 3100

Confidential Enquiry into Stillbirths and Deaths in Infancy (CESDI)

Chiltern Court
188 Baker Street
London
NW1 5SD

Cystic Fibrosis Trust

11 London Road
Bromley
Kent
BR1 1BY
Tel: 020 8464 7211
Fax: 020 8311 0472
Website: www.cftrust.org.uk
Email: enquiries@cftrust.org.uk

Down's Syndrome Association

155 Mitcham Road
London
SW19 9PG
Tel: 020 8682 4001
Fax: 020 8682 4012
Website: down-syndrome.org.uk
Email: info@down-syndrome.org.uk

Eclampsia APEC

Achon on Pre-eclampsia (APEC)
84–88 Pinner Road
Harrow
Middlesex
HA1 4HZ
Tel: 020 8863 3271

Helpline: 020 8847 4231
Fax: 020 8824 0653
Website: www.apec.org.uk
Email: info@apec.org.uk

Foundation for Study of Sudden Infant Deaths

Artillery House
11–19 Artillery Row
London
SW1P 1RT
Enq: 020 7222 8001
Helpline: 020 7233 2090
Fax: 020 7222 8002
Website: www.sids.org.uk/fsid/
Email: info@sids.org.uk

Health Service Commissioner for England (OMBUDSMAN)

4th Floor
Millbank Tower
Millbank
London
SW1P 4QP
Tel: 020 7217 4050
Fax: 020 7217 4000
Website: www.ombudsman.org.uk
Enq: Enquiries@ombudsman.gsi.gov.uk

Human Fertilization and Embryology Authority

Paxton House
30 Artillery Lane
London
E1 7LS
Tel: 020 7377 5077
Website: www.hfea.gov.uk

King's Fund

11–13 Cavendish Square
London
W1M 0AN
Tel: 020 7307 2400
Website: www.kingsfund.org.uk

La'Leche League of GB (LLLGB)

BM Box 3424
London
WC1N 3XX
Helpline: 020 7242 1278
Website: www.laleche.org.uk

The Maternity Alliance

(Educational Research Trust)
45 Beech Street
London
EC2P 2LP
Tel: 0171 588 8582
Website: www.maternityalliance.org.uk

The Meet-a-Mum Association (MAMA)

14 Willis Road
Croydon
CRO 2XX
Website: www.mama.org.uk

MIDIRS

9 Elmsdale Road
Clifton
Bristol
BS8 1SL
Tel: 01179 251791
Website: www.midirs.org

National Audit Office (NAO)

157–197 Buckingham Palace Road
Victoria
London
SW1W 9SP
Tel: 020 7798 7000
Website: www.nao.gov.uk

National Childbirth Trust (NCT)

Alexandra House
Oldham Terrace
Acton
London
W3 6NH
Helpline: 0870 444 8704
Breastfeeding line: 0870 444 8708
Info line: 020 8992 2616
Fax: 020 8992 5929
Website: www.nct-online.org

National Council for Voluntary Organisations

Regents Wharf
8 All Saints Street
London
N1 9RL
Info: 020 7713 6161
Fax: 020 7713 6300
Website: www.ncvo-vol.org.uk
Email: nvco@ncvo-vol.org.uk

National Deaf Children's Society

15 Dufferin Street
London
CE1Y 8UR
Tel: 020 7490 8656
Helpline: 020 7250 0123
Fax: 020 7251 5020
Website: www.ndcs.org.uk

National Health Service Direct Helpline

0845 4647

National Institute for Clinical Excellence (NICE)

90 Long Acre
Covent Garden
London
WC2F 9RZ
Tel: 020 7849 3444
Website: www.nice.org.uk

NMC Nursing and Midwifery Council

23 Portland Place
London
W1N 4JT
Tel: 020 7580 7642

National Organisation for Counselling Adopters and Parents (NORCAP)

12 Church Road
Wheatley
Oxfordshire
OX33 1LU
Tel: 01865 875000
Fax: 01865 875686
Website: www.norcap.org.uk

National Society for Phenylketonuria (UK) Ltd

NSPKU
PO Box 26642
London
N14 4ZF
Helpline: 0845 603 9136
Website: neb.ukonline.co.uk/nspku
Email: nspku@ukonline.co.uk

Royal College of Midwives

15 Mansfield Street
London
W1M 0BE
Tel: 020 7872 5110
Website: www.rcm.org.uk

The Royal College of Obstetricians and Gynaecologists

27 Sussex Place
Regents Park
London
NW1 4RG
Tel: 020 7772 6200
Website: www.rcog.org.uk

SANDS (Stillbirth and Neonatal Death Society)

28 Portland Place
London
W1N 4DE
Website: www.uk-sands.org

Sickle Cell Society

54 Station Road
Harlesden
London
NW10 4UA
Tel: 020 8961 7795/4006
Fax: 020 8961 8346
Website: www.sicklecellsociety.org
Email: sicklecellsoc@btinternet.com

TAMBA (Twins and Multiple Birth Association)

Harnott House
309 Chester Road
Little Sutton
Ellesmere Port
CH66 1QQ
Tel: 0870 121 4000/0151 348 0020
Fax: 0870 121 4001
Website: www.tamba.org.uk
Email: enquiries@tambahq.org.uk

Terrence Higgins Trust Lighthouse

52–54 Gray's Inn Road
London
WC1X 8JU
Info line 020 7831 0330
Helpline: 020 7242 1010
Fax: 020 7242 0121
Website: www.tht.org.uk

WHO

Avenue Appia
CH-1211 Geneva 27
Switzerland
Tel: +41 (22) 791 2111
Website: www.who.ch